The Acne Prescription

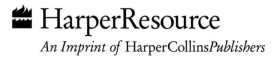
HarperResource
An Imprint of HarperCollins*Publishers*

The Acne Prescription

The Perricone Program
for Clear and Healthy
Skin at Every Age

Nicholas Perricone, M.D.

Line drawings copyright © 2003 by Alexis Seabrook.

Excerpt from *Woman as Healer* by Jeanne Achterberg copyright © 1990 by Jeanne Achterberg. Reprinted by arrangement with Shambhala Publications, Inc., Boston, MA (www. shambhala.com).

"Health Benefits of Yoga" by Trisha Lamb Feuerstein copyright © 2001 by Trisha Lamb Feuerstein. Used by permission of the author and the Yoga Research and Education Center (www.yrec.org).

This book is written as a source of information only. The information contained in this book should by no means be considered a substitute for the advice of a qualified medical professional, who should always be consulted before beginning any new diet, exercise or other health program.

All efforts have been made to ensure the accuracy of information contained in this book as of the date published. The author and the publisher expressly disclaim responsibility for any adverse effects arising from the use or application of the information contained herein.

The names of the patients in this book have been changed to protect their privacy. HarperCollins books may be purchased for educational, business, or sales promotional use. For information please write: Special Markets Department, HarperCollins Publishers Inc., 10 East 53rd Street, New York, NY 10022.

FIRST EDITION

Designed by Joy O'Meara-Battista

Printed on acid-free paper

Library of Congress Cataloging-in-Publication Data

Perricone, Nicholas.
   The acne prescription : the Perricone program for clear and healthy skin at every age / Nicholas Perricone.
      p.   cm.
   ISBN 0-06-018878-2
   1. Acne.   2. Acne—Treatment.   3. Skin—Diseases—Treatment.   I. Title.
RL131 .P467 2003
616.5'3—dc21   2003050943

03   04   05   06   07   RRD   10   9   8   7   6   5   4   3   2   1

To my patients of 15 years who have taught me as much as my medical school and residency. I thank you for the privilege of serving you.

CONTENTS

ACKNOWLEDGMENTS

Many people contributed to the success of this book, and I want to thank all of my friends and colleagues for their ongoing support of my work.

A very special thank-you to Anne Sellaro for her ability to turn visionary goals into concrete realities. Her matchless skills, creativity, enthusiasm, and tireless support enable me to bring my message to millions of people worldwide, for which I remain eternally grateful.

To the outstanding team at HarperCollins including: Jennifer Brehl, my very talented and hardworking editor; Shelby Meizlik, publicity superwoman; Kate Stark, marketing genius; Robin Bilardello and Andrea Brown for outstanding book jacket design; Megan Newman, editorial director extraordinaire; Jane Friedman, Cathy Hemming, and Steve Hanselman for friendship and support at the highest levels of the publishing world. I also want to thank the entire HarperCollins sales force for their outstanding work in seeing that my books are well stocked and prominently displayed in bookstores everywhere.

Special thanks also to: Dean Glenn Craig Davis, M.D., and the Michigan State University College of Human Medicine; Michigan State University President Peter McPherson; David Vigliano; Tony Tiano and Lennlee Melton; Kyle MacLachlan and Desiree Gruber; Kim Cattrall; the staff at NV Perricone M.D., Ltd.; the Public Broadcasting Service (PBS) and all of their member stations nationwide; Harry Preuss, M.D.; Christiane Northrup, M.D.; Mr. and Mrs. Richard Post; Marvin Josephson; Heidi Klum; Michelle Bega; Ally Bernstein and Casey Johnson; Jill Eisenstadt; Nicole Esposito; *I*village.com; the Colony Club; National Council of Jewish Women; the ESPY Awards; Cosmetic Executive Women (CEW); City of Hope; *In Style* Golden Globes Event; the Fifth Annual *Forbes* Executive Women's Forum; Fashion Group International; Possible Women sixth annual leadership conference; the Connecticut Intellectual Property Law Association; the Eli Whitney Award; Book Mania Event; Walter Camp Foundation; Karen MacKenzie; Larry DiNardis,

Jackie Koral, and friends at the University of New Haven; Ronald Hoffman, M.D.; the American College of Nutrition; the American Academy for the Advancement of Medicine; Hillary Clark; the Presidio San Francisco; Lippe Taylor; Sephora; Neiman Marcus; Saks Fifth Avenue; Henri Bendel; Clydes on Madison; Nordstrom; Trimmingham's; Craig Weatherby; Vincent Perricone; my children, Nicholas, Jeff, and Caitlin; Roger Rich; Ed and Elizabeth Walsh; Maria Verel; Dallas Hartnet; Bernadette Penotti; the Learning Society of Boston; the New York Learning Annex; RJ Julia; Fashion Group International; the staff and Guenter Richter, managing director of the St. Regis Hotel.

INTRODUCTION

Acne is a disease that can occur in virtually anyone at almost any stage of his or her life. Acne not only disfigures the face and body but can also leave profound, permanent scars on one's self-esteem. I know this first-hand, because in my teens through early twenties I suffered from acne. It was not until after my discharge from the army that I was fortunate enough to meet the man who would help me, Dr. Sidney Hurwitz, a highly regarded pediatric dermatologist. Dr. Hurwitz treated me with a then-experimental group of new drugs called retinoids. Much to my delight, the treatment was a success. But I gained much more than freedom from acne. Inspired by Dr. Hurwitz's dedicated work and compassionate care, I found an important life goal: to become a physician specializing in dermatology.

The Acne Prescription is a labor of love and of revelation. As you will learn, acne is a systemic inflammatory disease. Readers familiar with my work know that the three-tiered anti-inflammatory lifestyle is the cornerstone of my research and treatment methodology. If you follow it properly and faithfully, you can prevent or delay the onset of many diseases and degenerative conditions that begin at the cellular level.

I have tailored my three-tiered approach, which has helped so many people reverse the outward signs of aging, to help those suffering from acne. The good news is that it works for everyone—young *and* old, male *and* female. In my private practice I have helped clear acne in all types of people, including teenagers of both sexes, young mothers, middle-aged businessmen, thirty-something career women, and young male body-builders. What do they all have in common? Inflammation at the cellular level.

Because I spent so many years in a fruitless search for a treatment to clear my acne (before finally meeting Dr. Hurwitz), I am especially sensitive to the anger and frustration many of you experience in dealing with this disease. In *The Acne Prescription* you will learn how to take control of the onset and duration of your acne lesions. Most important, you will also learn how to prevent new lesions from forming.

If you follow my simple 28-Day Program of diet, exercise, and nutritional supplements and use the recommended topical anti-inflammatories, your acne should resolve without your having to resort to some of the more common, drastic measures that often produce unpleasant side effects. You will learn how to heal yourself from the inside out—and the only side effects you'll experience are clear, beautiful skin and a rejuvenated body and brain.

Thanks for accompanying me on this journey to empowerment. I welcome your letters and e-mails, which you may send to me at www.nvperriconemd.com.

Nicholas Perricone, M.D.
February 2003

1

The ABCs of Acne

1986 was a banner year for me. After many years spent undergoing rigorous medical training and testing, I was about to begin my private dermatological practice. I had received my medical degree from Michigan State University College of Human Medicine, followed by a one-year internship in pediatrics at Yale New Haven Hospital. I then completed a three-year residency at the Ford Medical Center in my specialty, dermatology, and was now ready and eager to begin seeing and treating patients. Dermatology—the diagnosis and treatment of the skin and its diseases—is one of those specialties that has patients of every age—from infancy to old age, and every point in between.

It is interesting to note that in my dermatological residency we spent very little time studying the causes and treatment of acne—one of the most prevalent yet difficult skin diseases to successfully treat. In addition to the physical disfigurement caused by the blemishes, acne can also leave deep scars on the psyche. Despite these facts, close to two thirds of our time was spent learning how to diagnose and treat other skin diseases. A full one third of the residency was spent learning how to perform dermatological surgery.

As a newly graduated dermatology resident with board certification, I opened a solo practice in Connecticut—where I quickly discovered that a large portion of my patients suffered from acne. I was comfortable treating my adolescent acne patients, as I myself had suffered from fairly severe acne that began around the time I turned fourteen and continued to plague me throughout my early and mid-twenties. I could empathize with the teenagers who came seeking my help; I had been there.

My Story

When I developed acne in my teens, I lacked the financial means to seek professional medical advice or treatment for it. I haunted the corner drugstore searching the shelves for remedies. About the best I could find were products that contained active ingredients such as sulfur in a tinted base—over-the-counter medicated cover-up creams. They helped a little at first but soon lost their effectiveness. By the time I reached college I finally began seeing a dermatologist. I was treated with a range of things—from ultraviolet radiation and oral antibiotics (such as tetracycline), to topical abrasive scrubs containing tiny bits of sand, followed by tinted hydrocortisone-based lotions. The doctor also performed what I called acne surgery. He used an instrument to actually unplug the affected pores. We continued these treatments for approximately six months, after which I felt that there was not enough improvement to justify the time, expense, and discomfort.

Following college graduation, I entered the army, where I had severe acne flare-ups during both basic and advanced training. The army, however, did not consider acne a disease worth treating, so there were no options open to me other than to endure the condition and bide my time.

After suffering an arm injury, I spent a few months in an army hospital. I finally had the opportunity to speak to a physician about my acne but was too embarrassed to bring it up. This was a tertiary care hospital; all around me were patients in need of acute or critical care. In the bed to the right of me lay a soldier who had been hit by AK-47 fire and whose arm bones had been shattered. To my left was a man with both arms in casts, suffering from severe burns and fractures sustained from enemy fire on his helicopter. Although my right arm was in a cast, what I was most concerned about was my acne!

After I was discharged from active army duty, I was once again employed (although I'd not yet decided to enter medicine). I immediately sought help from a dermatologist. I went through a number of treatments, none of which seemed to bring any relief, leaving me depressed and discouraged.

Vitamin A for Acne Relief

One lucky day, a friend of mine told me about Dr. Sidney Hurwitz, one of the first pediatric dermatologists in the country. Dr. Hurwitz was a true innovator who kept up with the latest dermatological developments and treatments. He was achieving greater results than just about anyone in dermatology at that time. Dr. Hurwitz had been a board-certified practicing pediatrician who had decided to enter a three-year dermatological residency program to become a dermatologist. Now that his specialties were both dermatology and pediatrics, he limited his practice to patients no older than sixteen. Although I was well over that age, I was determined to see him. I called Dr. Hurwitz, explained my situation, and asked if he would make an exception in my case. Much to my delight, he said yes.

During my first office visit I was very impressed with Dr. Hurwitz, both as a man and as a physician. He was brimming with incredible enthusiasm for his work, and I could see that he loved taking care of his patients. For the first time in more than a decade, I felt a genuine sense of hope and renewed optimism. After examining my face and cataloging the long list of my previous treatments, he asked me an intriguing question: "Have you tried vitamin A to treat your acne?"

In my ongoing search for a cure I had read about vitamin A and taken large self-prescribed doses of the supplement, but had not seen any effects. "I am referring to a new form of vitamin A that is applied topically—directly to the skin," he explained. "The University of Pennsylvania has been conducting extensive research utilizing vitamin A acid and has a product in early clinical trials." He then told me that Johnson & Johnson had licensed the technology. I was ready and willing to be a guinea pig, and I eagerly agreed to participate in the study. Dr. Hurwitz used this new product on me in combination with other topical and oral medications, and over a period of a few months, my face completely cleared.

In addition to the great joy and satisfaction I felt with my newly clear complexion, I also gained extensive firsthand knowledge of the latest and most effective acne treatments. This proved to be of great help to me in later years when I started my own practice. It was also a turning point in my life. It was Dr. Hurwitz's impressive dedication, skill, and thirst for knowledge that inspired me to follow him into dermatology.

As the number of my acne patients began to multiply, I was eager to help them on their way to an acne-free future. However, to my surprise, close to half of these patients were men and women (mostly women) in their twenties, thirties, and forties. The remaining half were adolescents. As I well knew from my own experience, adolescent acne is usually characterized by an oily complexion. Yet my older female acne patients often had dry, sensitive skin. However, as is still true, the vast majority of available topical acne medications were developed to treat teenagers who have typical adolescent oily skin, and contain ingredients that are actually drying and *proinflammatory*. This left me with few conventional treatment options for treating my adult patients. It also left me pondering the puzzle of why and how two such totally different skin types could suffer from the same disease.

While having oily skin might exacerbate acne, it is not the root cause. I knew this because during my residency program at Henry Ford Hospital in Detroit, Michigan, more than 80 percent of my patients were African American. African-American skin is typically rich in *sebaceous* (oil-producing) glands, yet African Americans suffer far less acne than other ethnic groups. It is interesting to note that acne in Africans is almost nonexistent, yet there are instances of acne among African-Americans although, as mentioned, less than other ethnic groups. Further, it is known that Native Americans had virtually no acne until their adoption of Western diets and intermarriage with other ethnic groups. What is clear is that there is some genetic component to acne. Obviously the Western diet plays a major role in acne development, a fascinating topic we will cover in later chapters.

Anatomy of a Lesion

In order to begin to treat acne, we must first learn some simple anatomy of the skin. Let's begin at the surface, called the *stratum corneum.* It is made up of dead, protein-rich cells known as *keratin,* which acts as a protective barrier for the underlying cells.

Just below the stratum corneum exists a layer of living cells, called the *spiny layer* because when these cells are viewed under the microscope, they appear to contain a series of little bridges. As we continue moving down through the *epidermis* (the outermost layer of the skin), we come to a layer known as the *basal cells.* The basal cells are constantly dividing and migrating toward the skin's surface and are the precursors to all of the layers we have just described. Simply stated, basal cells grow and divide. And as they move toward the surface of the skin they mature, eventually becoming the dead layer known as the stratum corneum. This maturation process of basal cells into the stratum corneum is called *keratinization.*

To understand the physical changes that cause acne, it is important to understand the microscopic processes that produce it. We all know that our skin has pores. Dermatologists refer to these pores as *follicles.* Many of us think of a follicle as a small hair (since we usually hear it being referred to as a hair follicle); however, the follicle could either contain a hair or it could be empty. Imagine the follicle as a tube, extending from the surface of the skin down into the *dermis,* or the skin layer beneath the epidermis.

This deeper layer of skin—the dermis—is made up of *collagen* and *elastin,* which support the surface of the skin and provide a home for blood vessels, nerves, and other cells. Directly beneath the dermis is a layer of fat that cushions and insulates the skin and contributes to the rounded look of a youthful face. The follicle (or pore) originates from the dermis as a tube. From this tube branch glands that resemble little clusters of grapes. These are the sebaceous (or oil) glands that produce an oily substance dermatologists call *sebum.* The sebum flows to the top of the tube (follicle), eventually to be secreted onto the skin's surface. (I should mention here that there is some debate among scientists as to whether sebum does or does not lubricate skin, but that is not important to our story.)

Now that we understand some of the basic anatomy of the skin, let's look at what actually causes acne. Most scientists believe that the primary cause of an acne lesion (commonly called a pimple) is something called *retention hyperkeratosis*. In reality the primary event is inflammation which then causes the retention hyperkeratosis. As we discussed, the surface of the skin, the top layer of the epidermis is called the stratum corneum. The dead cells of the stratum corneum, which contain a large amount of the protein keratin, are supposed to fall off the skin in a natural process called *exfoliation,* or *desquamation.* This stratum corneum also lines the inside of the follicle (tube). Scientists believe that if the inside of the follicle doesn't exfoliate properly, the keratin mixes with sebum, making it viscous and sticky, clogging the follicle. We will review in depth throughout the chapters and explain how inflammation causes the above chain of events.

Why doesn't acne make its first appearance before puberty? The answer to that is *hormones.* When we enter puberty, our body begins to produce *testosterone.* Testosterone breaks down into a substance called *dihydrotestosterone* (DHT) that stimulates the sebaceous gland to produce more sebum. For many reasons, this sebum begins the process of retention hyperkeratosis, or insufficient exfoliation within the follicle lining.

For a moment, pretend we could look down into that follicle. There we would see that the dead stratum corneum cells are not being carried away by the flow of oil from the sebaceous glands, due to the insufficient exfoliation. Instead, they remain inside the follicle where they form a sticky mass. Within a short time a bacterium, *Propionibacterium acnes,* begins to multiply rapidly, creating further inflammation within the follicle and surrounding skin. If new stratum corneum cells continue to be generated, but the dead ones are not exfoliating, the resulting condition is known as retention hyperkeratosis. The term "retention hyperkeratosis" simply means that the pore is retaining the stratum corneum cells, resulting in a clogged pore.

The dermatological term for this plug is *comedo* (plural "comedones"). When the comedo is initially formed beneath the epidermis, it is too small to be seen with the naked eye. At this point such a lesion is called a *microcomedo.* As it enlarges, it looks like a tiny white bump just below the surface of the skin. If you slide your finger over your skin you can often feel these small, hard bumps. As these lesions enlarge they grow from microcomedones into comedone*s* and then into other larger lesions—full-grown pimples.

And here is where a significant error has been made. To this day physicians and scientists erroneously believe that there are only two types of acne lesions which are categorized either as noninflamed or inflamed.

Inflamed Lesions and the Myth of the Noninflamed Lesion

Let's continue looking at the anatomy of acne lesions and their development for a clearer understanding of them.

The microcomedo ultimately evolved into a *closed* comedo, also known as a "whitehead." The other so-called noninflamed lesion is the *open* comedo, or "blackhead." In this case the oil and the still open follicle have been oxidized by the air, turning it brown or black. The blackhead also contains a pigment called melanin.

If this lesion is able to drain to the surface it will be resolved. The other possibility is that the comedo cannot drain, and inflammation moves from the invisible, molecular level, to the visible, cellular level. It develops into a *papule* and then finally into a *pustule,* which we refer to as a pimple. Visible inflammation can progress even further; that is the lesion can become deeper and more severe, resulting in a *nodule* or a *cyst.*

Scientists use a grading system to categorize the various stages of acne lesions.

Grade 1 comprises microcomedones and the comedones—the whiteheads and blackheads that are traditionally referred to as noninflammatory acne lesions.

Grade 2 is the papule—a small, pink, visibly inflamed bump that is tender to the touch and which conventional science recognizes as an inflammatory lesion.

Grade 3 is the pustule, a lesion with more visible inflammation than the papule.

Grade 4 is the nodule, a large, painful, solid lesion extending deep into the skin, accompanied by visible inflammation.

Grade 5 is the cyst—an inflamed, pus-filled lesion extending deep into the skin. This occurs when several nodules merge resulting in a giant lesion.

Now, let's take a closer look at the myth of the noninflamed acne lesion.

The accepted grading system outlined above is based on *visible* inflammation. Note that Grade 1 is considered noninflamed. Although we will be looking at the inflammatory process on a cellular level in another chapter, let's take a look now at some of the changes that occur to this so-called noninflamed acne lesion. To recap, here is the series of events that create a comedo. The follicle becomes clogged by dead cells that mix with oil (sebum), and thus does not exfoliate properly. Bacteria then begin to break down the sebum into fatty acids. The result is a micro-comedo which eventually will look to the naked eye like a little white grain of sand beneath the skin. The follicular wall, which is made up of cells, is stretched by this retention hyperkeratosis, and may then become a lesion that appears to be inflamed. Or the impaction may eventually work its way out, resulting in no visible inflammation. However, the so-called noninflamed comedo is actually producing proinflammatory chemicals called *cytokines,* which are invisible even under the microscope because their molecules are far too small to be seen.

At this point, bacteria have infiltrated the comedo (clogged pore), breaking sebum (oil) down into fatty acids, resulting in a condition known as *oxidative stress* in the surrounding cells. Oxidative stress is caused when free radicals (bad molecules) overwhelm the antioxidants, which are the natural defense system of the cell. This results in changes in the *redox status,* which is responsible for maintaining the fine balance of the cell by carefully and precisely controlling the balance between free radicals (bad guys) and antioxidants (good guys).

When the cell comes under oxidative stress, tiny molecules known as *transcription factors* are activated. When the transcription factor known as NfkB (nuclear factor kappa B) is activated, it goes to the nucleus of the cell where it turns on a gene that causes the cell to produce proinflammatory chemicals known as cytokines such as *interleukins* and *tumor necrosis factor alpha.* The inflammatory cytokines some of which are known as in-

On Controlling Germs

"By the end of the nineteenth century, the work of Lister, Pasteur, Koch, and other 'microbe hunters' led to the germ theory of disease and to knowledge of sepsis and antisepsis. Hospital procedures and sanitation dramatically improved.

"Even before the germ theory, another man—Ignaz Semmelweis (1818–1865)—was successful in learning to control the spread of puerperal (childbed) fever, caused by *Streptococcus pyogenes.* His is a long, sad story, representing the worst that can happen when one challenges the prevailing mode of thought.

"Semmelweis reasoned that dirty hands were the cause of puerperal fever. He noted that wards staffed by medical students had about 10 percent mortality rate due to fever, while those staffed by midwives had . . . 3 percent. . . . He also knew that medical students went straight from autopsy chambers to laboring mothers. They [the med students] never washed their hands, but wiped them, instead, on aprons already coated with body fluids.

"Semmelweis ran several experiments requiring students to wash their hands with soap and water and rinse them in chlorinated lime solution before entering the wards. With each study, the death rate dropped to less than 1.5 percent, only to return to the previous high levels when the [hand washing] procedures were curtailed.

"Semmelweis's work should have proven to be a boon to motherhood and life. Not so. His colleagues greeted his paper with jeers and scathing attacks on his character. They simply refused to believe that their own hands were the vehicle for disease. Instead, they attributed it to a spontaneous phenomenon arising from the 'combustible' nature of the parturient woman. Semmelweis's academic rank was lowered, his hospital privileges restricted. Despondent, he was committed to an insane asylum, where he died of blood poisoning, a disease not unlike the puerperal fever he had almost conquered."[1]

terleukins can act as messengers throughout the cell but they can actually leak out of the cell, where they trigger further free radical or oxidative stress. When this occurs, interleukin 1 makes keratinocytes sticky which results in formation of the microcomedo. In addition, interleukins can cause the breakdown of cells, allowing the migration of white blood cells to the area. Inflammation now becomes visible. Cytokines are tiny molecules of protein that are proinflammatory. Remember, they switch on inflammation at a cellular level. In its earliest stages—for example, a Grade 1 acne lesion—this inflammation is invisible. But left untreated, the inflammation will become visible in the form of retention hyperkeratosis and are too small to be seen under the microscope.

Scientists and physicians are certainly aware of the existence of proinflammatory cytokines, yet they still believe that comedones are non-inflammatory acne lesions. However, there are many factors that prove that both types of Grade 1 acne lesions are inflammatory lesions:

- An inflammatory cytokine, interleukin-1 triggered by stress, diet and other factors, causes abnormal exfoliation within the follicle making the cells known as keratinocytes stick together causing a comedone.
- The oxidative stress found in comedones triggers activation of the transcription factor NkB, which then produces cytokines.
- The fatty acids in the impacted follicle actually mimic molecules similar to a platelet-activating factor and act as messengers in the body to produce inflammation.
- The stretching of the follicular wall caused by the impaction results in a disruption of the cell plasma membrane, causing the release of *phospholipids,* which in turn are broken down into proinflammatory chemicals.
- Arachidonic acid levels are elevated in these disrupted cell walls, resulting in further release of proinflammatory chemicals such as *leukotrienes* B4.

Scientists have measured increased levels of inflammatory cytokines in the so-called noninflamed acne lesion.[2] And yet most scientists believe that there are *two* types of acne lesions, noninflamed and inflamed, because evidence of inflammation in the noninflamed acne lesion cannot be seen under a microscope.

Medical science has a long tradition of such misconceptions. The story of Dr. Semmelweis is a classic example. I have been a fan of public television for decades. One day I was watching my favorite PBS station, WNET/Channel 13, out of New York City. That day they were running a show featuring biographies of famous physicians. It was here that I first learned of the groundbreaking work of Dr. Ignaz Semmelweis.

The Inflammation Comes First

Thanks to my research into the causes of aging skin, I have learned a tremendous amount about inflammation and its connection to most disease processes, including wrinkling. And because my approach was so novel and different, (i.e., searching for ways to lessen and/or eliminate the inflammation at a cellular level, it would prove to be of tremendous help in my search for technology that would tackle the acne problem.

> "Even when all the experts agree, they may well be mistaken."
> —Bertrand Russell

As we have mentioned several times, dermatologists believe that the primary event in the formation of an acne lesion is a clogged pore called a comedo. They believe that this comedo is a noninflamed lesion because they cannot see the inflammation under their microscopes. But I must mention this again, in reality the inflammation always comes first and it is the inflammation that causes the clogged pore or comedo.

The following is so important that I must apologize for repeating it again, Interleukin 1, a cytokine that acts as a cellular messenger, can make the cells within the follicles sticky which results in a clogged pore. Remember when we eat foods that are proinflammatory or when we are under stress it can all lead to the introduction of interleukin-1.

Eyes Wide Shut

Dr. Semmelweis's colleagues could not believe that something they couldn't see could be causing such far reaching damage to these women who were giving birth. Now more than a century later, physicians are still refusing to believe in something they cannot see under the microscope.

More and more scientists from all disciplines are recognizing that inflammation is indeed a major contributing factor to aging, disease and its accompanying symptoms. A recent study which appeared in the Journal of Clinical Endocrinology and Metabolism (May 2003) affirms that two major markers of inflammation *"Insulin-like growth factor 1 and interleukin-6 contribute synergistically to disability and mortality in older women."* The authors conclude that "the joint effects of IGF-1 and IL-6 may be important targets for treatments to prevent or minimize disability associated with aging." My own research has shown that these two inflammatory markers play a significant role in acne as well.

Diet and its relationship to acne have similarly been denied. However, two studies that appeared in Archives in Dermatology in 2002, *Acne Vulgaris: A Disease of Western Civilization* and *Diet and Acne Revisited* confirm my long held assertion that diet is a critical factor in acne, aging and disease in general.

It is a tragedy that tens of thousands of patients—young and old, rich and poor—died because medical experts wouldn't believe what they couldn't see. And now, more than 150 years later, we are in the same situation. Modern-day physicians do not believe that inflammation is at the basis of the so-called noninflamed acne lesion—thus helping to ensure that they will never develop very effective therapies for this disease.

But this is just a small part of it.

When I was in medical school I found evidence that inflammation may be the basis of many diverse diseases—including heart disease, cancer, arthritis, autoimmune disease, even problems like Alzheimer's and Parkinson's. Probably the most controversial belief I hold regarding inflammation is that it is at the very *basis* of aging—in short, that aging is an *inflammatory disease.* Needless to say, most scientists and physicians are not terribly enthusiastic about this hypothesis. Why? Because inflammation cannot always be seen—even under the most powerful microscope.

Unlike the admirable Mr. Spock, we humans tend to let our emotions interfere with our logic. Physicians and scientists are perhaps among the most susceptible to this human frailty. When they do not agree for any reason with a radical hypothesis or nonconformist opinion about the cause of a disease, they not only vehemently reject it they also exhibit irrational, emotional, and angry behavior toward the message *and* the messenger. As you might conclude, this has a deleterious effect on the progress of science and medicine.

> "The trouble with the world is that the stupid are cocksure and the intelligent are full of doubt."
> —Bertrand Russell

Let's look at the inflammatory cascade that *is* visible and that scientists *can* see. This will help us to understand why they call these inflammatory acne lesions.

As mentioned earlier, these lesions (Grades 2, 3, 4, and 5) are described as the papule, pustule, the nodule, and the cyst. And yes, these particular lesions exhibit visible signs of inflammation. Under a microscope, white blood cells are rampant in and around the impacted follicles, where they secrete enzymes that further break down the cells, signaling the classic inflammatory response. When a large number of white cells (called *polymorphonuclear* cells) congregate in a localized area of the body in response to the presence of bacterial infection, they form a visible entity that we call pus. Pus is present in both papules and pustules; if the process occurs deep within the follicle, a nodule is formed; if nodules merge, a cyst is formed.

When viewed by the naked eye in a clinical exam, redness and/or swelling—accepted signs of an inflammatory response—are apparent. Under the microscope, it may be seen that white blood cells are migrating toward the area of the impacted follicle, and secreting enzymes that further break down the cells in that area, exacerbating the inflammatory response.

If you are wondering why I continue to drive home this point, it is because things that are invisible *can* hurt you and cause serious problems, very much like the germs that killed all those new mothers in the maternity hospital. If we consider the noninflamed acne lesion an inflamed lesion, and understand the function of cytokines, we can control these lesions with anti-inflammatories. How? First we can approach it systemically, by altering our diets and changing our lifestyles to decrease inflammation on a cellular level. Second, we can do it topically through the use of creams and lotions that contain powerful anti-inflammatory ingredients.

We can put the fire out before it becomes visible—before we look in the mirror and discover an inflamed acne lesion. Why is this so important? After all, what's the big deal about a few pimples, really, other than the insult to our vanity? Well, if acne is allowed to continue unchecked, treated only when it becomes visible, the invisible inflammation at the cellular level results in white blood cells surrounding the follicle which destroy tissue. Once this tissue is broken down and then repaired by the body, we end up with either *atrophic* scars (deep, indented scars resulting from collagen loss) or *hypertrophic* scars (bumpy scars made up of an excess of collagen). Even worse, very large lesions may result in huge scars known as *keloids,* which are extremely difficult to treat. The good news is that armed with a little knowledge we can prevent acne lesions from ever reaching this stage. Acne is a systemic inflammatory disease; to successfully prevent and treat it we must adopt strategies proven to reduce inflammation in the body.

The Three-Tiered Perricone Program for Reducing Inflammation

Those of you who have read my first two books, *The Wrinkle Cure* and *The Perricone Prescription,* are familiar with my three-tiered approach (diet, nutritional supplements, and topical applications) to reduce inflammation at the cellular level. In those books I explained the connection between inflammation, aging, and age-related diseases. In this book we'll look at the relationship between inflammation and acne. Like wrinkles and many signs of aging, acne is an inflammatory disease, and it *can* be controlled.

Read on to learn more about the causes of acne—and what you can do to be acne free for life!

2

Traditional Treatment of Acne— Past and Present

One of the great paradoxes of traditional medicine's treatment of acne lies in its long-established and time-honored treatments of choice. As with my discoveries in treating aging and aging skin, I can never resist challenging the prevailing wisdom—especially when it appears to spring from a false premise. Such is the case with the treatment of acne. Acne is a systemic *inflammatory* disease.[1] And yet the traditional treatments of choice are proinflammatory!

Before I outline for you my three-tiered anti-inflammatory program for the treatment of acne, it is worthwhile to take a good, hard look at conventional treatments—and their shortcomings.

Back to the Future

Believe it or not, the acne treatments first developed by dermatologists way back in the 1800s differ little from the over-the-counter medications you'll find in your neighborhood drugstore today. Applying sulfur results in drying of skin and this was standard therapy in the 1800s. The sulfur was often accompanied by other irritants, which helped loosen the impactions within the clogged pores.

During the 1940s and 1950s dermatologists also used mixtures containing sulfur, which were known as drying lotions. Some of these lotions included antibacterial ingredients, to assist in efficacy. Clearasil, a still-popular sulfur-containing over-the-counter acne treatment, was one of the products I tried as a teenager. Sulfur medications work initially, but they tend to lose their efficacy with prolonged use.[2] It has been shown that the skin quickly acclimates to the active ingredients, whose purpose is to irritate the blemish, causing it to peel and expose the impaction.

In the 1800s another interesting discovery was made regarding acne. Thanks to the microscope, scientists were able to examine acne lesions much more closely than ever before. And, one of the things they found was that bacteria were present in the lesions. Thus, they deduced that these bacteria were a cause of acne. But it was not until the development of antibiotics in the late 1940s and early 1950s that antibacterial treatment was used in the fight against acne. Penicillin, the first available antibiotic, was tried as an acne therapy, but appeared to have no therapeutic effect. Scientists surmised that although penicillin circulated in the bloodstream it did not get into the skin. Fortunately, other antibiotics (such as tetracycline) were subsequently discovered that *did* demonstrate activity in the skin. Early studies revealed that acne patients who were treated with oral tetracycline showed some improvement, making this the preferred acne treatment for several decades. Other antibiotics that were also popular were erythromycin and clindamycin. While clindamycin (the original name of which was Cleocin), showed some efficacy, its possible side effects included diarrhea and colitis, an inflammation of the gastrointestinal tract. (It should be noted that in a number of severe cases, the colitis proved to be fatal.)

In addition to oral antibiotic therapy, antibiotics may also be applied topically. The antibiotic (such as erythromycin or clindamycin) is mixed with alcohol, penetration enhancers, and emollients, and applied to the skin once or twice daily. This treatment has been shown to be effective and, when used in conjunction with other topical medications, such as *benzoyl peroxide,* results are greatly improved.

Benzoyl peroxide is a popular acne medication that is available in both over-the-counter and prescription strengths. Its effectiveness comes from its antibacterial properties and its ability to act as a peeling agent. It also appears to limit the secretion of certain oils that contain fatty acids, which contribute to acne flare-ups. I have found that many of my acne patients respond well to a combination of benzoyl peroxide and topical antibiotics. In certain cases, I may also prescribe retinoids.

Vitamin A Acid (Retin-A)

Another important acne treatment was developed in the late 1960s and introduced to the market in the early 1970s. This treatment is *vitamin-A acid,* also known as Retin-A. Retin-A acid is the acidic form of vitamin A. When applied topically, it normalizes the desquamation inside the follicle, thereby helping to loosen the patches of dead material. As I mentioned earlier, I was introduced to Retin-A by acclaimed dermatologist Dr. Sydney Hurwitz, and this treatment had a dramatic positive affect on my acne. Of course Retin-A, or Retin-A acid, like benzoyl peroxide and other topical treatments, is quite irritating. Most patients experience *tremendous amounts of inflammation* during the first few weeks of therapy.[3] This may sound contradictory as anyone who has applied Retin-A knows that the skin gets red and inflamed from the treatment.

This has been an ongoing problem with traditional acne treatments; they are extremely irritating—in fact, they are proinflammatory. And as we know by now, acne is an inflammatory disease. This is particularly important when treating adult patients, especially women, who do not have the oily skin of the adolescent acne sufferer. Until now, adult patients have been stuck in a classic Catch-22 treatment situation; the cure was similar to the problem—both were inflammatory!

Accutane

The breakthroughs achieved by using topical vitamin A acid also led to another oral therapy, this one made from a compound belonging to the same retinoid class as Retin-A. This compound is called isotretinoin (13-cis-retinoic acid) and is known by the trade name *Accutane.* When taken for approximately four to five months, Accutane has been proven to be an extremely effective treatment for a severe form of acne known as cystic or nodular acne. In fact, for those suffering from severe cystic acne, Accutane has proven to be nothing short of a miracle.

But Accutane, a prescription medication, has a number of possible serious side effects that are similar to those resulting from large doses of vitamin A. Among Accutane's potential side effects are dry, peeling skin; a sudden inability to see in the dark (so night driving can be dangerous); intracranial pressure, which can lead to permanent loss of sight, or in rare instances, death. Another possible side effect is inflammation of the liver, which can be detected by blood tests. For this reason, periodic blood tests are performed on patients undergoing Accutane treatment. Fortunately, I didn't see this side effect very often in my patients who used Accutane unless they were also consuming alcohol or taking other prescription medications. Elevated triglycerides are another possible side effect of Accutane. This too can be detected by blood tests. Once the Accutane treatment is ended, most patients' triglyceride levels return to normal.

According to the detailed information posted on the FDA (federal Food and Drug Administration) website, Accutane can cause severe birth defects if taken by pregnant women. It can also cause miscarriage, premature birth, or death of the baby. For this reason, women of childbearing age who take Accutane must not be pregnant or become pregnant during treatment or for three months after discontinuing treatment. There has also been a link between taking Accutane and mental depression and suicide. If your physician prescribes Accutane, consider increasing your daily intake of essential fatty acids and be sure to eat salmon once a day. Probably the most common side effect of Accutane that I saw in my practice was severe dry skin, lips, and nasal passages, which resulted in flaking skin, chapped lips, and nosebleeds. Due to the potentially very serious side effects of Accutane, I strongly recommend that you consult your dermatologist and also refer to the FDA's website page devoted to Accutane: www.fda.gov/cder/drug/infopage/accutane/medicationguide.htm that provides a comprehensive look at the risks and benefits of this treatment.

Research into various retinoid treatments for acne is ongoing. Other topical retinoids are now being used that tend to be less irritating to the skin, although I have not observed this in my practice when prescribing these alternative retinoids.

Other prescription treatments include oral contraceptives, which have proven effective for women with acne. Oral contraceptives may normalize the hormonal changes, helping to prevent the hormonal surges that can aggravate acne.

Alpha hydroxy acids, such as *glycolic acid* (derived from sugar cane), are another over-the-counter acne treatment. They work by helping to increase shedding of skin cells. This helps to clear the impaction within the follicle. Glycolic acid also acts as a powerful antibacterial and anti-inflammatory agent. If we look at the molecular structure of glycolic acid and compare it to ascorbic acid (vitamin C), we see that their structures are similar. Vitamin C also has anti-inflammatory properties, which we will discuss in depth in the chapter that focuses on the newer treatments for acne (Chapter Four). In this chapter we will look at the use of targeted nutritional supplements and the importance of good nutrition in the treatment and prevention of acne. And you will learn that the myth that diet and nutritional supplements don't have an impact on acne is just that—a myth.

In addition to oral and topical compounds, acne patients have been subjected to many procedures in search of a cure. Back in the early 1900s, German physicians treated their acne patients with X-ray therapy. Initial studies showed this type of therapy to be extremely effective. This led to X-ray therapy being used on tens of thousands of patients, who later developed multiple skin cancers and cancer of the thyroid from the radiation. To make matters worse, at a later date, dermatologists who tried X-ray therapy found that it had no effect—good or bad—on their patients' acne.

Another acne treatment of long-standing yet dubious merit is ultraviolet radiation. We receive ultraviolet radiation naturally from the sun. However, starting in the 1950s and continuing through the 1980s (and, occasionally, today), physicians administered artificially generated ultraviolet light treatments to their acne patients. Like the X-ray treatments, this, too, has proved to be an unfortunate therapy; as we now know, ultraviolet radiation increases our risk of cancer and accelerates the aging process. And, to top it off, it is not particularly effective in the treatment of acne.

That's not to say that all the traditional therapies are duds. An effective form of treatment that has very few side effects is *cryotherapy*—targeted freezing of the skin. Physicians either rub dry ice onto the skin or apply liquid nitrogen directly to the acne lesions. The downside is that to ensure optimum effectiveness, cryotherapy should be administered daily, which makes this form of treatment impractical for the average patient.

Another acne treatment is a procedure known as acne surgery. The physician uses a small instrument that presses down upon the acne lesion, forcing out the impaction. This treatment must be performed regularly. However, insurance companies do not cover this mode of treatment, so it is not very popular. Nor, based on my own experience, is it all that effective.

After a quick rundown of some of these traditional treatments it becomes apparent that:

- They are not particularly effective, yet carry risks.
- They work but are not practical due to treatment frequency, prohibitive cost, etc.
- They do work but have potentially serious side effects.
- They are very effective but are proinflammatory.

Retin-A and many over-the-counter treatments can be irritating. In fact, these treatments actually make the acne worse before—maybe—making it better.[4] In particular, these treatments can be a disastrous choice for adult patients, whose skin is very different from that of adolescents. Yes, they may help the acne—but at what price? Dry skin? Accelerated aging?

Two New Therapies with Promise

Some physicians are treating acne with a specific wavelength of laser light that focuses on a pigment known as *prophyrin* (a pigment in the skin), which is produced by the *Propionibacterium acnes* bacteria. These prophyrins are very sensitive to laser light of 410 to 420 nanometers; laser light at this intensity can destroy the bacteria, which, in turn, decreases levels of fatty acids and cytokines (such as interleukins)—resulting in decreased inflammation. Some experts believe that the heat produced by the laser light may also be therapeutic.

Another new therapy currently being tested employs radio waves, which actually heat the dermis (the lower portion of the skin), without burning the surface. The surface of the skin is first rapidly cooled with liquid nitrogen, after which a measured dosage of radio waves is applied. Proper implementation of this therapy requires the administration of an anesthetic to the skin; and so patients undergoing this treatment must be under a physician's care. Although this treatment is very new, it shows considerable promise and may soon be another viable alternative acne therapy you may want to discuss with your dermatologist.

Anti-inflammatory Treatments for Acne

Treating acne as the systemic, proinflammatory disease that it is opens up entirely new treatment options. My research and the experiences of untold numbers of acne sufferers have shown that many traditional acne treatments are ineffective at best, harmful at worst. As a physician I was taught: "first do no harm." Taking this premise to heart, I have developed a program that will help prevent and heal acne lesions *from the inside out as well as from the outside in.* By embracing the anti-inflammatory lifestyle, getting adequate sleep, drinking enough water, and learning how to decrease your stress levels, you can and will dramatically affect the way your body reacts to this disease.

Armed with this knowledge, I have devised a three-tiered program to treat acne. Tier one is the anti-inflammatory diet. Tier two is targeted nutritional supplements with anti-inflammatory properties. And Tier three is anti-inflammatory topical treatments. I've used this program with hundreds of patients in my private practice—and it works. Read on and learn how you can integrate the Perricone Anti-Acne Program into your life, to *treat and prevent* this emotionally and physically disfiguring disease.

3

The Many Faces of Acne

Acne is a heartbreaking, disfiguring disease that can occur in people of almost any age, regardless of gender and skin type. Dermatologists know that the age range of two to six years is considered the acne-free zone, during which *acne vulgaris* (common acne) rarely occurs. Even newborns can develop acne, possibly due to hormonal changes that occur as the fetus develops. Although it has not yet been definitively determined why elderly people do not develop acne, it may have to do with the decrease in hormonal activity that comes with advancing age.

Despite the fact that acne can strike at nearly any age, it is firmly ensconced in our collective consciousness as an adolescent disease. For decades, both acne treatments and advertising have been almost exclusively directed at this age group. Television and magazines are rife with images of teenage angst—adolescent boys and girls peering in their mirrors as they attempt to cover up unsightly blemishes.

However, as any dermatologist can tell you, this is only half the story. Acne affects almost as many women in their late twenties, thirties, and forties as it does adolescents. My waiting room is frequently filled with acne patients both adolescent and adult, eager for treatment. Although acne can and does affect adult males, the majority of acne patients are women. This may be due to the fact that society tends to put more focus on women's faces, but as the modern man increasingly pays more attention to his self-image, we will no doubt be seeing more men seeking acne treatment. Since adult skin is much different than adolescent skin, treatments that are effective for adolescent acne are usually unacceptable for adults, particularly adult women. We must develop a whole new bag of tricks to treat acne in the adult female. Each woman is also unique in many different ways—and these differences may all converge to bring about the onset and flare-ups of acne.

Getting the Red Out

No, we aren't talking about eye drops! The red we are referring to here is the redness of a skin condition known as *rosacea*. Rosacea is a chronic skin disorder that appears to be more common in women than in men. For years it has been commonly confused with acne. It usually appears in middle age or later. According to an excellent information website, www.rosacea.org, an estimated 14 million Americans have rosacea and many don't know it. Although we don't know the cause, rosacea is an inflammatory condition characterized by dilated capillaries on the skin's surface. Patients also complain of easily blushing and flushing of the face. Other symptoms include skin thickening, pimples and bumps, and persistent redness, mostly on the forehead, nose, cheekbones and chin. Following the anti-inflammatory diet found in this book is very important for rosacea sufferers. Many experts recommend avoiding hot spicy foods, hot beverages, extreme hot and extreme cold temperatures, sun exposure, alcohol, and any irritating skin treatments or products (including facial peels and alpha hydroxy acid products). See your dermatologist for treatment. Make sure you follow my anti-inflammatory diet which contains essential fatty acids and supplement with flax and borage oils. Also, make sure you keep your skin very clean—do not wash with just water. Use a gentle but thorough cleanser morning and evening (preferably containing alpha lipoic acid) to remove bacteria. Topical alpha lipoic acid can decrease the redness associated with rosacea that cannot be improved by prescription medications such as Metronidazole. Rosacea has also been treated in the past with antibiotics. Thanks to the power of the anti-inflammatory diet, these treatments oftentimes prove unnecessary.

The Critical Difference: Lisa's Story

Lisa is typical of many of my women acne patients. During our first consultation, I asked her to tell me about her daily life. This is because many factors—both internal and external—affect a person's skin. From childhood, Lisa had been blessed with beautiful, clear, flawless skin. Her fair, porcelain-like complexion is accompanied by naturally blond hair and blue eyes. She had scrupulously avoided excess sun exposure to prevent the premature lines and wrinkles she had observed on the face of her mother, an ardent sportswoman who was perpetually tanned.

As a high-profile broker for an international real estate firm, Lisa's appearance was a great asset. Her glamorous job involved extensive travel, marketing and selling some of the world's most luxurious homes—from Manhattan penthouses to London townhouses, Malibu beachfront estates to Loire Valley chateaux. At the age of thirty-five, Lisa was approaching the pinnacle of her career. But with great success can come increased stress, and I could see evidence that Lisa was experiencing a great deal of stress.

Out of the blue, her face had suddenly begun to erupt in serious and unsightly acne lesions. She'd come to me, desperate for help.

"I'm at my wit's end, Dr. Perricone," Lisa confided. "What is happening?"

"Lisa, believe it or not, you are experiencing a classic case of adult-onset acne," I explained.

Like many of her peers, Lisa thought it extremely unlikely that someone of her age, who had not suffered from acne during her teen years, could now develop a skin condition that appeared to be acne. In fact, she did not believe that it *could* be acne.

"The fact is, Lisa, close to half my acne patients are adults—and the majority of those are women," I explained. I proceeded to take Lisa's full medical history and ascertained that she enjoyed excellent health. Laboratory studies taken by her gynecologist indicated normal levels of hormones. Lisa also exercised regularly. However, she admitted that recently she'd been experiencing higher than normal stress levels.

"It's strange, Dr. Perricone. I usually thrive on the high-pressure, high-stakes game of the luxury real estate market, but lately I'm tense and anxious and find it difficult to unwind at the end of the day. And now this! I'm really stressed about these breakouts, and I'm desperate to do something about them." She went on to mention that the lesions seemed to flare up about a week before her twice-monthly sales goals and forecast meetings, and would persist for days.

Hormones and Acne—the Link

Lisa is a classic example of the female acne patient in her late twenties, thirties, or forties. Although acne is the same systemic inflammatory disease in both adolescents and adults, the precipitating events leading to its onset differ greatly between teens and adults.

Changing hormone levels affect the onset of acne. We know that the sebaceous glands can be stimulated by hormones to produce sebum. The male hormones (androgens) stimulate oil production by binding to a special receptor on the oil gland. An enzyme present in the oil gland breaks down these androgen-type hormones, such as testosterone, into a more powerful hormone called dihydrotestosterone (DHT).[1]

Doctors differ in their opinions about the role of estrogen in acne. Some physicians believe that as levels of the hormone progesterone decrease in women as they age, the estrogen comes to predominate, and may cause a problem. Other physicians believe that estrogen is helpful, because the increase of hormones like estrogen that bind up the testosterone also reduces the production of testosterone and other androgens.[2]

But simply measuring the testosterone level in blood does not tell us much because some testosterone is bound to a protein, and only the testosterone that is not bound has an effect on the oil glands. We must also bear in mind that a woman's ovaries can produce androgens (which are male hormones). In addition, androgens can be produced by the adrenal gland (a small gland that sits on top of the kidney), which also produces something called *dehydroepiandrosterone* (DHEA). The androgens produced by a woman's ovaries and the DHEA produced by her adrenal glands can then affect the oil glands, causing them to convert the androgens into a more potent form, via the enzyme 5-alpha reductase type 1.

Studies have been conducted to ascertain how many women with acne actually have abnormal levels of circulating hormones. The results of one study showed that about half the women did; another study indicated that the incidence was much higher—between 60 and 90 percent. I think that those numbers are high; most of the women I have examined possess normal androgen levels.

Put in layman's terms, the male hormones, called androgens, stimulate the oil glands to produce more sebum, and that may contribute to the development of acne in some people.

Scientists have devised ways of treating acne by altering hormone levels. One of the inexpensive ways for a woman to do this is to use oral contraceptives. By taking a birth control pill, a woman can increase the levels of proteins that bind the male hormone testosterone. Women who took a prescription oral contraceptive called Ortho-tri-Cyclen, had levels of unbound testosterone almost 50 percent lower than the levels in women who took other birth control pills. However, I don't recommend oral contraceptives as a first line of treatment because of their other risks and side effects. In fact, Lisa felt that the oral contraceptives she was taking seemed to make her skin worse.

Physicians have devised additional methods to influence hormones that are known as *anti-androgen chemicals.* One of these, *spironolactone,* is actually a diuretic, or water pill. Spironolactone binds to the androgen receptors, preventing the conversion of testosterone to the more powerful hormone DHT. But its side effects may include increased urination, abnormal menstrual periods, weight gain, breast tenderness, dizziness, and headaches. Diuretics can also drain the body of potassium, another dangerous side effect. *Flutamide,* another androgen blocker that has been used to treat male pattern baldness, has not been successful in treating acne and should not be used for this purpose.

Lisa, like approximately 80 to 90 percent of my female acne patients, reported that she experienced flare-ups when she was premenstrual. The sebaceous glands can be affected by the hormonal changes that occur during the midcycle of the menstrual period. While there is controversy regarding the effects of estrogen and progesterone on acne, we do know that altering the hormone status to prevent hormonal surges can be therapeutic to some women. I believe that estrogen acts as a natural anti-inflammatory and exerts a systemic anti-inflammatory effect that is beneficial to the skin.

I was not surprised to learn that Lisa complained of flare-ups that seemed to be caused by her oral contraceptive. Many oral contraceptives have an androgenic effect on the body, causing it to become more acne prone. The newer oral contraceptives have been designed to avoid the androgen effect. Yet, while some physicians believe that taking oral contraceptives is helpful to women acne sufferers, I believe that the most effective and safest course of treatment is to control hormonal surges and acne flare-ups through an anti-inflammatory diet and with anti-inflammatory nutritional supplements. As will be shown later in this book, these methods work to heal and balance the body naturally and effectively—and without negative side effects.

All Shook Up: Stress, Women, and Acne

Stress is a proven precipitator of acne at any age.[3] Yet here is another arena in which the adolescent and adult differ greatly. As we'll discuss a little later in this chapter, young people are able to bounce back from the effects of *cortisol,* a stress hormone, within a matter of hours. On the other hand, when the release of cortisol is triggered in adults, it can circulate through their system for days, exacerbating acne flare-ups.

It is sad but true that acne often rears its ugly head at the most inopportune times. Ask anyone who has had acne, and he or she will confirm that it has an uncanny knack of flaring up just in time for that special event—a first date, important job interview, or wedding! This happens far too frequently to be chalked up to bad luck or coincidence. Believe it or not, this is actually good news. It means that instead of being a random occurrence, there is an identifiable physiological cause of acne flare-ups: *stress.*

Of all the physical conditions we experience, stress is the most deadly. Many circumstances create stress in our daily lives. Arguments with family, friends, or colleagues; not enough sleep; worry; working too hard or even playing too hard can all create stress. Weekend warriors who try to make up for a week spent sitting at a desk by spending hours in strenuous physical activity raise their stress levels to an unhealthy degree. Any activity that is practiced in excess can lead to a stress response. This is extremely important to remember if you hope to control your acne flare-ups.

To understand the stress response we must learn a little bit about the adrenal hormones. Any form of stress, whether emotional or physical, results in the activation of the stress response in our bodies. It is the body's survival mechanism, and has been since humankind's earliest days. For example, thousands of years ago, when humans lived in caves, a simple stroll to the watering hole might mean an unpleasant encounter with a wild and hungry animal. Such a confrontation would cause an immediate surge of adrenaline to course through the body, accompanied by a release of the stress hormone cortisol into the bloodstream. This team of hormones kick starts the body, energizing it to get out of that stressful situation— sometimes with seemingly superhuman speed. When adrenaline and cortisol kick into action, blood sugar and amino acid levels rise, providing energy at the cellular level to activate the body's fight or flight response.

This was a very good thing when the fight or flight response came in handy for the occasional chance meeting with a saber-toothed tiger. But when you fast-forward to modern society, with its constant, daily stressors—from traffic jams to college exams—a problem arises. The protective fight or flight mechanism is forced to work overtime, resulting in constantly elevated levels of cortisol.

Those of you who are familiar with my work in the anti-aging field know that elevated levels of cortisol are very destructive to the body.[4,5] Elevated cortisol levels cause an increase in blood sugar, which in turn causes an instantaneous response from our cells as they enter an extreme proinflammatory mode. You may be asking yourself, "How can what goes on in my adrenal glands have an effect on my acne?"

As I have mentioned before, acne is a systemic, inflammatory disease. According to Webster's dictionary, systemic means "of or pertaining to the general system, or the body as a whole." Simply put, everything you do—from eating to exercise, undergoing stress to sleeping (or not!)—has an impact on your acne.

Cortisol—the Death Hormone

Cortisol is the one hormone that actually increases as we get older. We are all familiar with cortisol, because a derivative called cortisone is used in topical and systemic medications and has been part of the pharmacological arsenal for years. Cortisol is essential; it enables our internal systems to maintain stability and stay in balance during acute forms of stress, such as fear, physical trauma, and extreme physical exertion. When it is needed during periods of stress, cortisol is produced by the body in the quantities necessary to combat that stress. However, a problem arises when cortisol is present for long periods of time and in excess quantities. When we measure the cortisol levels of a young person under stress, they rise rapidly, but within a few hours as the stress is relieved, they decline to normal. However, when we measure cortisol levels in older people, the levels rise rapidly during stress but tend not to return to normal for days. Since cortisol levels continue to increase with age, a sixty-five-year-old has far higher levels of cortisol circulating throughout his system than does a twenty-five-year-old.

Large amounts of cortisol are toxic when they circulate in our system for prolonged periods of time. Our brain cells, or neurons, are extremely sensitive to the effects of cortisol. When cortisol is circulating at a high level, it causes the brain cells to die. That is why brain shrinkage is associated with senility in old age. Excessive amounts of cortisol can destroy the immune system, shrink the brain and other vital organs, decrease muscle mass, and cause thinning of the skin which results in prominent blood vessels. In the anti-aging field, cortisol is known as the death hormone because it is associated with old age and disease.

Reprinted from *The Perricone Prescription*.

The Missing Link—the Neuropeptide Connection

There are other connections between acne and stress besides the endocrine or hormonal connection. There is a direct link between the brain, and the action of nerves in the skin which can affect both the onset and course of acne. Scientists now know that the brain can cause the release of chemicals in the nerves in the skin, especially those close to the oil gland. The chemicals released by these abundant nerve endings in facial skin are called *neuropeptides*.

A neuropeptide that is getting a lot of attention, especially in the realm of acne, is Substance P (SP). Substance P can affect the sebaceous gland by making it more active and also by affecting its growth.

It is interesting to note that the skin of acne patients has a much greater number of these Substance P containing nerves than the average person.

It is also interesting to note that there are several hundred neuropeptides functioning in our body and they are intimately involved with the immune system and the inflammatory response. We know that neuropeptide secretion precipitates inflammation in many skin diseases, including acne. Therefore when an individual is psychologically stressed, this stress causes the release of Substance P from nerves. The result? An inflammatory cascade and the production of cytokines such as Interleukin's 1 and 6.

As we know, Interleukin-1 is a very important factor in the formation of the basic acne lesion. Since we now know that acne is both initiated and made worse by psychological stress, we now know that neuropeptides, such as Substance P, are the missing link.

In summary, neuropeptides can increase the size and activity of the sebaceous gland, which then produces more sebum than is observed in the skin of the acne patient. In addition, neuropeptides can initiate an inflammatory response by the production of cytokines such as Interleukin 1, which may be directly responsible for the formation of the basic acne lesion, the microcomedo. By preventing normal exfoliation within the follicle, we can see that the increased oil production by the follicle will then be trapped by sticky cells causing a clogged pore, which then can be secondarily infected by bacteria, amplifying the inflammatory reaction.

Thus we can see the brain/acne connection is a powerful one, mediated by neuropeptides with the final common pathway, as always, inflammation.

Scientists have been puzzled for years because there are so many factors that influence the onset and course of acne, they know hormonal effects are important; that bacteria play a role. Genetics and other precipitating agents contribute to acne. Now the mystery is solved because whether it is endocrine, psychological, excess oil in the skin, the final common pathway of initiation and progression is *inflammation*. It is important that scientists understand that the inflammation comes first and that acne is a systemic inflammatory disease which is manifested clinically in the skin.

As you know from my previous books and television lectures, diet is critical in controlling inflammation and inflammation is also the final common pathway for the mechanisms of aging and age related diseases. We can now step out of the dark ages with this knowledge just as the discovery of the microscope lifted us out of the darkness that Dr. Semmelweis faced in trying to convince his fellow physicians of the invisible cause of infection. Now our scientists and physicians, especially dermatologists trained in microscopic diagnosis, a specialty called dermatopathology, must understand that there are invisible factors that cause acne and other diseases that cannot be seen by their microscope.

Mars versus Venus: Androgens and Acne

When blood sugar and insulin levels rise, whether resulting from poor diet or excess stress, the body experiences a serious increase in inflammatory chemicals at the cellular level. This, in turn, causes inflammatory diseases such as acne to worsen—often dramatically. Cortisol and other adrenal steroids can act as androgens, and stimulate the sebaceous glands, resulting in an acne flare-up.

Another negative effect of elevated blood sugar is the storage of

Inequality of the Sexes

Although men are affected by stress and proinflammatory cortisol response, women undergo a double whammy—the proinflammatory cortisol-sugar-insulin connection *and* the effect of male-type hormones in their bodies. Men are not adversely affected by high levels of androgens in their systems in the same way women are, as androgens are male hormones. Women are susceptible to adrenal hormone stimulation because most of a woman's androgens are synthesized in the adrenal glands. The stimulation of the oil glands brought on by proinflammatory responses results in the changes we discussed earlier, including clogging of pores and increased secretion of proinflammatory fatty acids, which release the chemical messengers known as cytokines. Thus, the proinflammatory fire is fed.

body fat, especially around the abdomen due to its unique effects on certain receptors in that area's fat cells. This particular type of body fat is known as visceral fat, and it puts the body at greater risk for cardiovascular disease than fat stored in other areas of the body. In addition, when insulin levels are elevated, the body is less able to mobilize fat for energy production, resulting in a decreased ability to get rid of excess body fat. High insulin levels put a lock on body fat, making it very difficult to lose weight.

There are other factors in addition to stress that can release cortisol. Insufficient sleep causes cortisol levels to rise, and these levels will remain elevated for a full day following a poor night's rest. You may also notice that you crave carbohydrates the morning after a sleepless night. This is because elevated cortisol levels precipitate a rise in blood sugar, resulting in an insulin response, which triggers a rapid *drop* in blood sugar.[6] To compensate, many people binge on carbohydrates to counteract the process. But this only results in further inflammation of the cells, triggering or worsening an acne flare-up. Remember: the key to controlling and preventing acne breakouts is to keep blood sugar levels on an even keel. The roller-coaster ride of up and down, down and up only serves to exacerbate acne flare-ups (as well as many other degenerative conditions).

Elevated cortisol levels also contribute to acne flare-ups by stimulating the sebaceous glands, acting very much like other androgens. All of us have craved junk food following a particularly stressful event. In fact, there were many news stories after the September 11 attacks, reporting that these types of foods were wiped off the shelves of New York City stores. Again, the same mechanism as discussed above kicks in—cortisol is elevated, blood sugar is raised, an insulin response is triggered, resulting in that roller-coaster dive in blood sugar—and the body craves sweets and carbohydrates. Simultaneously, fats and amino acids are mobilized, in anticipation of the fight or flight syndrome, and the body experiences additional cravings—this time for salty foods.

Thus, elevated cortisol levels start a vicious cycle that is extremely dangerous not only to your overall health but also to your skin. If you are serious about preventing and treating acne, you must have a strategy to keep cortisol levels low.

Keeping Cortisol Under Control

In addition to following the anti-inflammatory diet and taking targeted anti-inflammatory nutritional supplements, you can incorporate these simple strategies into your daily life to guard against the cortisol roller coaster:

· **Get good, adequate sleep**—six to eight hours of uninterrupted sleep every night.

· **Minimize stress**—whenever possible, avoid stress-inducing situations.

· **Cut out coffee!** Coffee contains a number of organic acids that affect blood sugar and cortisol levels. This is *not* due to the caffeine. For example, you can drink a cup of decaffeinated coffee at 8 A.M., and your cortisol levels will still be measurable at 10 P.M.—the same as if you had drunk regular coffee.

· **Take time for yourself**—Set aside fifteen or twenty minutes a day for meditation or prayer. It is a well-established fact that people who do this have significantly lower cortisol levels than those who don't.[7,8] Proven long-term benefits include clear skin, a healthier immune system, and prevention of age-related diseases such as diabetes, cancer, and cardiovascular disease.

· **Yoga**—Yoga is an outstanding stress-reducing discipline as well as being of enormous benefit to overall fitness. See Chapter Seven for a series of basic yoga exercises to get you started.

· **Think green**—Substitute green tea for coffee. The benefits of green tea are many.[9-12] Many former coffee drinkers who switch to green tea report weight loss of up to ten pounds in just six weeks. While green tea does contain caffeine, it also contains a substance called theanine, which counteracts the negative effects of caffeine. Theanine protects the brain by preventing excitotoxity, which can cause irreversible damage to brain cells. Theanine is a natural mood elevator. Green tea also contains powerful antioxidants called polyphenols that are also excellent anti-inflammatories. Green tea prevents the absorption of fat, which in turn helps keep excess body fat under control.

An anti-inflammatory diet is of the primary importance in decreasing cortisol levels. In addition to all of the don'ts put forth in this chapter, there are a number of dos (get enough sleep, drink green tea, make time for yourself, etc.) that we must not ignore.

In addition to those dos listed above, do make sure there are plenty of essential fatty acids in your diet; they can decrease cortisol levels. This is so important that I mention it throughout this book. One of the most effective and delicious ways to do this is to eat a lot of wild Alaskan salmon. Canned salmon provides the same benefits as fresh; almost all canned salmon is from Alaska, but be sure to double-check the label.)

Other sources of essential fatty acids include avocados and nuts, particularly almonds, hazelnuts, pecans, Brazil nuts, and macadamia nuts.

Flaxseed oil is an excellent source and can be found in health food stores and some pharmacies. However, if you take a few moments to grind fresh flaxseed and sprinkle it on your morning oatmeal or yogurt you'll be in for a wonderful surprise. Flaxseed has a delicious nutty flavor and is loaded with the same omega-3 essential fatty acids that are found in salmon. In addition, flaxseed contains *lignans,* which have antitumor properties. Flaxseed is also high in fiber, which has been shown to help prevent certain forms of cancer (colon and breast) and aid in the prevention of coronary disease, when taken in the appropriate quantity (between 25 and 30 grams of fiber per day).[13] If you add just one quarter cup of ground flaxseed to your diet per day, it will provide approximately eleven to twelve grams of fiber. Store your flaxseeds (available in the refrigerated section of your health food and whole food stores) in the freezer to keep them from going rancid. For more recommendations on good food and tips for healthy eating and clear skin, refer to Chapter Four.

Getting Lisa on the Program

While Lisa was fascinated by my explanation of the stress-acne link, she was slightly skeptical of the great faith I placed in the anti-inflammatory diet. She had long subscribed to the popular opinion (one much touted by traditional dermatologists) that diet plays no role in acne—either for good or ill. This led me to ask her a simple question about her coffee intake. Lisa confessed that she drank between four and six cups of coffee daily, starting first thing in the morning and continuing throughout the day. No wonder she had trouble sleeping!

Here was the perfect opportunity to illustrate the direct link between cortisol levels, coffee intake, and lack of sleep. I outlined the process to her. Once Lisa understood this concept, I was confident her skepticism would fade—along with her jittery nerves and anxiety.

Lisa also revealed that she never drank water—in fact, she drank nothing that did not contain caffeine or sugar . . . and she preferred beverages that contained both. This dangerous habit was making a direct contribution to her acne. Although Lisa was generally healthy, she was well on her way to serious medical problems unless she changed her diet. In many ways, Lisa's sudden onset of acne was a wake-up call.

When I examined Lisa's skin I noticed it was fairly similar to that of most of my adult female acne patients. Her skin was on the dry side, and I suspected that her low-fat diet and severely low water intake were the principal cause. She had several inflamed papules along her jawline and chin. Several small patches of discoloration indicated previous deep lesions. I also noticed some mild redness, or *erythema,* which ended abruptly just below the jawline.

I asked Lisa what she was doing to treat her acne. She told me she had recently purchased an over-the-counter cleanser for acne-prone skin, which had been recommended by her neighborhood pharmacy. However, she found that it was causing her skin to become even drier than usual, and inflammation—which is common among women with Lisa's skin type—was visible.

Lisa's reaction was a perfect illustration of the difference between adolescent and mature skin. Her skin, which was already on the dry side, could not tolerate a strong, over-the-counter acne cleanser, which was devised with the oily skin of the adolescent acne sufferer in mind. The average adolescent skin can easily tolerate topical antibiotics, benzoyl-peroxide, and retinoids with no ill effects. But for Lisa, these treatments—which fill pharmacy shelves—result in marked redness and, possibly, burning of her sensitive skin.

As I examined Lisa's face, she explained that she enjoyed working out at the gym, as well as jogging and running outdoors, weather permitting. I asked her if she noticed any changes in her acne following physical exertion. Lisa admitted that prolonged workouts tended to trigger new acne flare-ups, whether the workout was at the gym or park. It all comes back to cortisol, I explained. Extended exercise results in a bodily stress reaction, elevating cortisol levels. This, in turn, aggravates acne. I counseled Lisa to moderate her exercise regimen to help control acne flare-ups.

Lisa's intense travel schedule also added to her stress. Flying between countries and time zones upset her internal clock. Over the years I have found that patients subjected to regular time zone changes usually experience acne flare-ups.

After the physical exam was completed, Lisa and I discussed her dietary habits and discovered that too much coffee was only the beginning! Lisa, like so many of my women patients, followed an extremely low-fat diet. Lisa's father had had a heart attack at age sixty, and her family had a history of cardiovascular disease and high blood pressure, which prompted her physician to recommend her strict low-fat regimen. However, as I have said time and again, low-fat and nonfat diets are extremely unhealthy. In fact, strict adherence to these diets can actually worsen acne and increase the risk of cardiovascular disease.

I asked Lisa to outline her average daily diet. She told me that breakfast usually consisted of a low-fat muffin and cup of coffee; lunch was a green salad without dressing and a small container of nonfat yogurt. Dinner varied, depending on whether she was at home or on the road, but she tried her best to stick to low-fat and nonfat foods.

Interestingly, the one "bad" food Lisa confessed a weakness for was chocolate. She said that whenever she gave in to her chocolate craving her acne worsened. Here I was able to give her some good news: Chocolate is actually an excellent food. It is high in antioxidants, and although it contains high levels of fat (which vary depending on the cocoa content), it is not the dangerous proinflammatory type of fat. Some chocolate is about 30 percent fat, mainly from cocoa butter, which contains about 60 percent saturated fatty acids (35 percent stearic acid and 25 percent palmitic acids) and about 40 percent unsaturated fatty acids (chiefly oleic acid). The negative effects on Lisa's acne were not from the chocolate. It was the sugar in the chocolate that aggravated the acne. I recommend chocolate that is 85 percent cocoa—as long as you don't eat too much, you'll reap the health benefits of chocolate and satisfy your craving.

I walked Lisa through the ill effects of her usual food choices after giving her a brief overview of the glycemic index—a one-to-one hundred scale that rates foods according to their impact on blood sugar levels, with one being the lowest and one hundred the highest (equaling the increase in blood sugar level that results from eating table sugar). I recommend avoiding foods that have a glycemic index rating higher than fifty. (For the most up-to-date information regarding the glycemic index ratings of various foods, check www.mendosa.com/gi/htm). For example, Lisa's morning muffin and coffee caused a spike in her blood sugar insulin levels resulting in a burst of inflammation. This had a negative impact on her acne as well as her overall health.

Lisa, like so many women, was eating a seriously protein-deficient diet. Protein is critical for cellular repair, and while she was not yet showing visible ravages of a low-protein diet, she was pushing the envelope. I told her that if she continued down this low or nonfat, low-protein dietary path for an extended length of time, she would soon look and feel at least ten years older than her actual age. In addition, her acne would be exacerbated—she'd have wrinkles *and* acne at the same time.

As we'll learn in Chapter Four, acne sufferers must learn how to regulate their blood sugar, keep it on an even keel day and night to avoid a chronic inflammatory state brought on by the up-and-down swings triggered by high glycemic foods. The best way to learn how to do this is to follow the Three-Day Nutritional Face-lift that I originally developed to rejuvenate aging skin. (See *The Perricone Prescription*.) The thousands of success stories shared with me by women and men attest to the far-reaching health and beauty effects on everything from arthritis to acne. I asked Lisa to begin with the three-day program before starting on the full 28-day regimen.

Although I always treat acne with a three-tiered approach (diet, nutritional supplements, and topicals), I held off starting Lisa on topical anti-inflammatories. I felt that it was critical to get her going on the anti-inflammatory diet and dietary supplements first—to begin treating her acne systematically, from the inside out. We made her next appointment for two weeks away, which would give her system time to adjust to its revised dietary regimen. I would then start her on some of the newer anti-inflammatory topicals, but first I wanted her to witness firsthand the all-important connection between food and her acne flare-ups. I gave Lisa a thirty-day supply of nutritional supplement packets that include the nutrients I recommend for acne-prone patients; she was to take one packet once daily at breakfast.

Although Lisa was highly motivated to adhere to the program, there were two areas in which I had serious reservations: coffee and water. Would Lisa be able to kick her coffee habit? And would she drink at least eight to ten glasses of water per day? Both these things were critical to the success of Lisa's acne treatment. As I expected, she was reluctant to give up coffee. However, the acne was so upsetting to her that she was willing

The Joy of Chocolate

While it is a long-held myth that chocolate causes acne, in reality chocolate not only tastes good, it is good for you, too.

Chocolate has numerous health benefits. In fact, about the worst thing you can say about chocolate is that it is often combined with high levels of sugar and trans fats. However, if you choose chocolate that contains 85 percent cocoa (read the label), you will be getting the supremely sweet benefits of chocolate without ingesting too much sugar. You may have to look a little harder to find this type of chocolate, certain chocolate specialty stores (such as Lindt) carry this product.

Just a few of chocolate's health benefits include:[14,15]

· Chocolate contains high levels of phenolics—powerful antioxidants that fight the cell damage that leads to chronic conditions such as cancer and heart diseases.

· Chocolate boosts levels of endorphins and serotonin—the brain's feel-good chemicals—when combined with the right amounts of sugar (i.e., very little) and (good) fat.

· Dark chocolate contains high levels of chromium, a substance that has been proven to control blood sugar.

So go ahead, indulge a little. Your brain, your body, *and* your sweet tooth will thank you for it!

to try. I suggested that she brew a large pot of green tea and drink it throughout the day. Green tea is also very refreshing as an iced beverage, especially when you add fresh lemon juice.

I stressed again the importance of drinking eight to ten glasses of water a day. I instructed her to visualize the water flushing out the toxins in her acne nodules. I also suggested that she keep bottles of spring water at her desk, by her bed, in the car, in her briefcase, by her gym bag, so she wouldn't conveniently forget all about it.

I also gave Lisa a daily journal in which she was to record her food and beverage intake, her moods and emotions, and the changes she noticed in her skin. Taking time to do this every day would help keep her motivated and on track. "Lisa," I promised, "you will feel and look better than you ever have if you start—and stick to—this program. Over the next few weeks, you can expect an elevation in your mood, an increase in your energy levels, and improved, sound sleep. Your brain will be sharper, your mind quicker, and work performance will improve. Most important, your stress levels will drop—and your skin will clear up." Lisa left in a buoyant mood, promising to call me in three days with a progress report.

Lisa's Turnaround

When Lisa called with her three-day progress report, she sounded enthusiastic and motivated. She had loved the immediate, visible results of the three-day program and couldn't wait to get started on the 28-day plan.

Three weeks later Lisa was sitting in my office. This time, however, she looked terrific and was fairly bubbling over with energy. She told me she felt fantastic—inside and out. And, best of all, she reported that she had kicked the coffee habit and found, to her amazement, that she now had more energy than when she was on caffeine.

Lisa had lost six pounds—"effortlessly," she enthused—since beginning the anti-inflammatory diet with nutritional supplements. As a result of keeping her blood sugar levels at a low, even keel, she was no longer experiencing up-and-down fluctuations in her energy levels, and her mood level stayed elevated throughout the day. In fact, she said, she felt wonderful. "The constant anxiety I used to feel seems to have disappeared."

But she was happiest about the appearance of her skin. Her acne flare-ups had lessened; the redness and irritation had decreased. As an added bonus, the chronic undereye bags and dark circles were greatly improved; she was finally getting a good night's sleep, every night. In fact, she said, her friends and colleagues had noticed the difference in her appearance and attitude and were eager to learn her secret.

I asked Lisa how she felt about the affect of her new lifestyle on her acne.

"Dr. Perricone, it's like magic," she said. "The lesions I have are resolving much more quickly than before. I just went through the midcycle of my menstrual period and didn't get the usual flare-ups. Even when my acne finally clears up for good I'll continue with the diet and supplements."

It was now time to introduce Lisa to the new topical agents. These would help continue her transformation without irritating her sensitive skin, as they worked synergistically with the anti-inflammatory foods and supplements. I explained that while many traditional acne medications work through their anti-inflammatory properties, they are also irritating (e.g., certain antibiotics act as anti-inflammatories, as do some traditional treatments such as Retin-A, salicylic acid and alpha hydroxy acid), my treatments are unique in that they contain patented anti-inflammatory substances that are vitamin or nutrient based.

Lisa's topical treatments included a cleanser containing anti-inflammatories (including DMAE, a nutrient found in fish), medicated toner pads, and a topical gel product that contains alpha lipoic acid, a powerful anti-inflammatory. I also gave Lisa a cover-up cream that contains therapeutic levels of DMAE, alpha lipoic acid, and glutathione, which could be used as a spot treatment to resolve lesions quickly—often overnight. Other active ingredients in Lisa's topicals included tocotrienols, an especially potent form of vitamin E, and vitamin C ester, a special fat-soluble form of vitamin C that rapidly penetrates the skin and has an anti-inflammatory effect on acne lesions.

Although these topicals are highly effective, they are nonirritating, which was very important to Lisa's sensitive skin. I advised her to stay on the program for four weeks, after which she should report back to me. I reminded her to continue drinking eight to ten glasses of spring water a day, to stay away from coffee, and continue to get a full 8 hours sleep every night. She told me that since starting the program, she was sleeping extremely well. She had moderated her exercise regimen to avoid triggering an acne flare-up. Finally, she confided that keeping the journal had been a huge help; she loved looking back and tracking the progress she'd made from day one.

Pregnancy and Acne

As we know, hormones can have a profound effect on acne. And women who are pregnant undergo intense hormonal fluctuations that can cause distressing acne flare-ups. To illustrate this, I'd like to share the story of one of my patients, Carmen.

When twenty-nine-year-old Carmen came to see me, she was angry, frustrated, and depressed. A beautiful woman of Hispanic descent, she had been plagued by adult acne for the past few years. The acne had been so severe that it had disfigured her lovely face, leaving scars and pits. A medical history revealed that she had been under a dermatologist's care for the past three years and had undergone both systemic and topical treatments, including the oral antibiotic minocycline, and the topical treatments benzoyl peroxide, Retin-A, and Cleocin solution (a topical antibiotic). Carmen had fairly oily skin, probably due to her Hispanic background. Even so, she found the topical treatments excessively drying and irritating at times, forcing her to discontinue the medications for week-long periods to allow her skin to recover.

When Carmen decided to become pregnant, her physician took her off all medications approximately six weeks prior to conception. I confirmed the wisdom of her doctor's decision, as I do not believe women should use oral or topical medications during pregnancy.

Carmen was now eight weeks pregnant. For the past four to five weeks out of the eight, she had been experiencing severe acne flare-ups. What could she do? she asked. The medications that had helped—despite their irritating side effects—were no longer an option.

I reassured Carmen that acne flare-ups are quite common during the first trimester of pregnancy. After the first three months, hormones readjust and the acne usually begins to resolve. I put Carmen on a well-balanced anti-inflammatory diet to help alleviate her acne; I knew it would give her the "from-the-inside-out" help she needed and would pose no threat to her developing fetus. In addition, I told her the good news: skin usually clears by the second or third trimester. However, I warned Carmen that the acne could return approximately two to three months after she gave birth, as a result of further hormonal changes. At that time, should the acne recur, we could discuss adding two more tiers to her treatment: anti-inflammatory supplements and anti-inflammatory topical medications.

Inflammation, Acne, and the African American

Alexa, a law professor at a New England university, did not develop acne until she was in her thirties. Alexa is African American and her dermatologist had placed her on a regimen similar to Carmen's, which included systemic and topical treatments—the oral antibiotic minocycline, and the topical treatments benzoyl peroxide, Retin-A, and cleocin solution (a topical antibiotic). Although the benzoyl peroxide helped somewhat with the breakouts, it turned Alexa's complexion an ashy gray. "I need your help, Dr. Perricone," Alexa said at our first consultation. "It seems I am trading one problem for another!"

Alexa was hopeful that I might have some alternative treatments that would work without unattractive side effects. She had also caught parts of my PBS specials on TV and was hoping that I might have some nutritional advice on how to improve her skin. In addition, Alexa confided that she experienced bouts of extreme fatigue.

After learning that Alexa's diet was carbohydrate-heavy and protein-light, I gave her a copy of the 28-Day Program and suggested she give it a try. I was very confident that I could help Alexa, but first I needed to dispel a very common myth in dermatology, and that is that darker-complected patients have *less sensitive* skin than the lighter-skinned northern Europeans. Actually the reverse is true as we examine African-American skin. In fact, one of the biggest problems experienced is a hyperinflammatory response in the skin to the slightest injury. Thus a single acne lesion will often result in the formation of an atrophic (indented) scar or a hypertrophic or keloid scar larger than the actual lesion itself. This occurs because the cellular response to injury in African Americans results in the greater production of pro-inflammatory chemicals and collagen-damaging enzymes. I explained to Alexa that her skin was very sensitive. She needed to follow a gentle, non-irritating regimen because it is critical that inflammation be prevented and aggressively treated in this skin type.

I have mentioned many times in my books and public television programs that the skin is a complex organ that perfectly reflects the changes taking place inside of our bodies. It is logical to assume that this hyperinflammatory response to injury takes place in all of the vital organs in the African American. This explains why they experience a higher incidence of high blood pressure, heart disease, stroke, diabetes, and some forms of cancer. The three-tiered anti-inflammatory approach to health and beauty is absolutely critical to the health and well-being of African Americans.

I gave Alexa the topical treatments containing alpha lipoic acid, DMAE and glutathione and cautioned her to cleanse gently—no scrubbing or abrasive cleansers.

One month later a new Alexa arrived at my office. "I don't know how to thank you, Dr. Perricone," Alexa enthused. I could see that her face literally glowed with health and radiance. It's not just the clear and radiant skin," she continued, "I feel like a kid again, just brimming over with energy!" Alexa had followed the anti-inflammatory 28-Day Program carefully and it had rewarded her by resolving her acne and restoring her energy levels. Additionally, Alexa's skin had responded beautifully to the gentle yet effective topical antioxidant anti-inflammatories. The ashy grayness was gone, replaced with a beautiful, even skin tone. I cannot ever emphasize enough how rewarding these kinds of success stories are to me—in fact I don't know who was more delighted—me or Alexa!

Cosmetics and Acne

It is a widely known fact that another major precipitator of adult female acne is cosmetics.[16] Why else would so many cosmetic companies herald their products with the rallying cry *noncomedogenic!* (a fancy way of saying "won't clog pores")? However, despite using cosmetics containing noncomedogenic ingredients, many women do end up suffering from acne. I always make it a point to look at the ingredients in my female patients' cosmetics, because many beauty products contain acne-inducing substances. These ingredients notwithstanding, it should be noted that the anti-inflammatory diet will greatly reduce susceptibility to comedogenic agents. And I am happy to report that the majority of my adult female patients who follow the antiinflammatory diet are so happy with the resulting increase of radiance in their skin that they no longer need to wear foundation.

Working with adult female acne patients has taught me a great deal. Their unique endocrine system and physiology, lifestyle habits, hormonal stages (from normal menstrual cycle to pregnancy to pre- or peri-menopausal and postmenopausal), cosmetics usage, and stress all contribute to acne in adult women. If you suffer from adult-onset acne, I urge you to adopt the anti-inflammatory lifestyle. Follow the 28-Day Program, take the appropriate nutritional supplements, and use the recommended topicals. Avoid coffee, excess alcohol, and tobacco, as well as sugary and starchy foods. Exercise in moderation, practice stress-relieving and relaxation-inducing techniques, and give yourself the gift of a good night's sleep.

This is the foundation of my program: good old-fashioned common sense coupled with up-to-the minute medical information. Every day I receive letters and e-mail messages from my patients and readers, sharing stories of their happy experiences on the Perricone Program. Like them, you, too, can say good-bye to acne forever—and enjoy a happier, healthier, more productive life in the process.

4

The Three-Tiered Perricone Anti-Acne Program— Tier 1: The Anti-Inflammatory Diet

Food Does Make a Difference

If you open any dermatology textbook to the chapter on acne, or pick up one of the popular books on acne written by dermatologists, you will find it emphatically—and unequivocally—stated that diet has no effect on acne. You will learn that eating sugary foods—such as candy, cookies, and cakes—or fried foods—such as potato chips, onion rings, and French fries—makes no difference at all as far your acne is concerned. This "fact" is stated with great emphasis and authority and has been the dermatologist's company line for decades. Naturally you would assume that hundreds of clinical studies on the subject had been conducted; how else could the scientific world have reached this unanimous conclusion? Well, you would be wrong! This misconception is based on just a few poorly designed and (knowing what we now know) obviously flawed studies.

   This assumption is representative of the many mistakes to be found in most acne textbooks. In addition to the misinformation regarding diet and acne that dermatology residents are taught is the myth of the noninflammatory acne lesion. You will remember from Chapter One that acne lesions are classified as either noninflammatory or inflammatory. However, acne is an inflammatory disease and *all* its lesions are inflammatory, regardless of whether the inflammation is visible under the dermatologist's microscope or not.

The prevailing wisdom is that the foods we eat have no effect on the systemic disease of acne. Food is the fuel that allows the body's organs (the largest of which is the skin) to perform at optimum levels. A poor diet full of proinflammatory foods will cause the body to break down and age prematurely, and will leave it susceptible to numerous diseases. Put aside scientific acumen—this is just plain common sense.

So where did this so-called prevailing wisdom come from and why is it held as a sacred cow to practitioners of an entire medical specialty? Thirty-odd years ago a small group of dermatologists enlisted two groups of teenage acne sufferers and gave them specially manufactured candy bars. One group received candy bars that contained high amounts of chocolate. The other group received candy bars that contained high amounts of vegetable oils. The dermatologists then observed both groups for a thirty-day period. Because these candy bars were prepared with or without chocolate, and with or without vegetable oil, while maintaining the same caloric value, it appeared—and was claimed—that the study was controlled.

Using common sense, one can quickly see the flaws in the study's design—even if one has no scientific background.

Let's examine the most glaring, obvious flaws.

1. First of all, there is *no mention* of the teenagers' diets at the beginning of the study. Were they chocoholics? Was fast food a dietary staple? The relevant questions are as varied as they are endless—and not one of them was asked.
2. The teenagers already had acne. Therefore, the introduction of the candy bars into the diet had no bearing on what *causes* acne—the unique set of conditions that existed for each individual and contributed to the onset of the disease. Under these circumstances, the most the dermatologists could hope to discover was what impact, if any, these two different types of candy bars had on the teens' *existing* acne.
3. The physicians had *no idea* what else the teens were eating during the study! To my way of thinking, this alone is a staggering deficit

of critical information. This critical variable was not even considered, making the use of the term "controlled study" absolutely false. In fact it is patently absurd.

As might be expected, neither group of teens showed any change in their acne after eating these candy bars for a solid month.

And so, thanks to a poorly designed and deeply flawed study, we have one of the greatest and most-often perpetuated myths in dermatological history! To add insult to injury, as the myth was propagated in classrooms and textbooks, generations of dermatologists were hampered in their ability to access all of the potential therapies for treating acne. Millions of acne sufferers were deprived of the basic knowledge that what they ate had everything to do with the onset and course of this disease.

As my patients and readers know, I am no stranger to challenging the status quo if it seems illogical, dangerous, or a combination of both. After close to two decades of treating acne patients, both adolescent and adult, I have seen firsthand the role of diet in *treating and preventing* acne. And my patients have told me time and time again that what they eat does make a difference in the onset and course of their acne.

I have often asked my colleagues if their patients ever claim that the foods they eat—or don't eat—make a difference in their acne. While they admit that this happens frequently, their attitude remains skeptical. If, I've been told, a patient states that he or she has found a food that really seems to clear up their acne, they condescendingly tell them to go ahead and stay with it "as long as you think it makes a difference"—a preemptory pat on the head bestowed as the doctor will reach for his prescription pad.

In my experience, the majority of my peers categorically believe that greasy foods such as French fries are not a contributing factor to acne. When asked why, the invariable answer is a reference to the aforementioned study and the fact that candy bars containing large amounts of vegetable oil had no effect on acne. From this, other erroneous conclusions are drawn: foods like pizza and sugared, carbonated beverages play no role in acne.

However, not all dermatologists believe that diet has no role in acne. Some forward-thinking dermatologists who acknowledge the link between diet and acne put their patients on an extremely low-fat, high carbohydrate diet—banning all fats and oils, good and bad. Forward thinking, yes, but still wrong. The dangers of this diet cannot be emphasized enough—in terms of acne and in relation to overall health, as will be explained in detail later in this chapter.

About the only concession some dermatologists make regarding the role of food and acne is regarding iodine. They concede that foods that contain iodine can exacerbate acne. Iodine is proinflammatory. In fact, large amounts of it can induce acne in anyone. People who have a propensity to iodine sensitivity may experience more rapid acne flare-ups when they ingest iodine. If this sounds like you, cut down on foods that are high in iodine.

The consensus among most dermatologists is that genetics, not diet, is the most important contributing factor to acne. This theory fails to hold water, however, when we consider that whole groups of genetically related people have *zero incidence* of acne in their native countries. Yet, once they come to the West or begin to follow a western diet, acne suddenly appears! Certainly there are other factors that contribute to acne, and I will cover some of the external factors at the end of this chapter. But first I will introduce you to the power of the anti-inflammatory diet and its incomparable ability to prevent acne and treat existing flare-ups.

The Anti-inflammatory Diet

Let food be thy medicine, thy medicine shall be thy food.
—HIPPOCRATES

Let nothing which can be treated by diet be treated by other means.
—MAIMONIDES

Our lives are not in the lap of the gods, but in the lap of our cooks.
—LIN YU-'TANG

Many of you may be familiar with my three previous books and public television specials in which I talk about the importance of the anti-inflammatory diet in preventing disease and maintaining youthful and beautiful skin, regardless of chronological age. However, I think it is important for new readers to understand the scientific foundation of my philosophy. Inflammation is at the basis of many diverse disease processes in the body, ranging from cancer to heart disease, acne to Alzheimer's, diabetes to the aging process in general.

We can all form a mental image of inflammation—for example, the boiled-lobster look of bad sunburn or the red, swollen thumb that results when we accidentally hit it with a hammer or catch it in a door. However, when I speak about inflammation I am referring to the *entire spectrum* of inflammation. This spectrum ranges from the mildest form of inflammation found on a cellular or molecular level to its strongest. But even low-grade inflammation, invisible to the naked eye, is very serious. Although it cannot be seen or felt, it is active in our cells every day, gradually damaging our vital organs, resulting in disease, aging, and eventually death.

I first came to this conclusion while in medical school, during my study of various disease processes under the microscope. I observed that inflammation was present in many disease processes. When I questioned my professors about this finding, they summarily dismissed my queries, stating that the inflammation was merely a by-product of the immune system and not a causative factor.

Rather than diminishing my interest in following this line of reasoning—that inflammation actually plays a role in the development of disease—I became more intrigued. I noted that inflammation was uniformly seen in the presence of cancer, and again I was told that this was *in no way* related to the cause of cancer. Instead, I was told again, it was simply a by-product of the immune system. I thought this odd for two reasons. First, many cancers proliferate because they avoid the immune system. Second, precancerous lesions also show evidence of inflammation.

In addition, when I looked through the microscope at the lesions seen in cardiovascular disease, *inflammation was always present.* Interestingly, inflammation was also present when I viewed aging skin through the microscope—yet young, disease-free skin showed *no signs of inflammation.* As I continued with my research, my belief was strengthened to a certainty beyond any doubt that inflammation was at the basis of these diseases. As a physician I made it my goal to find therapeutic approaches to prevent and control inflammation.

Long before attending medical school, I became interested in nutrition. Upon my discharge from the army I suffered from fatigue, yet my doctor could find no physical reasons to explain my chronic tiredness. This inspired me to look for alternative ways to regain my strength and energy. I began studying the work of many nontraditional nutritional experts such as Adele Davis and Linus Pauling. Their work inspired me to start taking nutritional supplements while still in my early twenties, a practice I have continued to the present day. I found that by following their dietary recommendations and nutritional supplement recommendations, my energy increased tremendously and my general health improved, as did my athletic performance.

By the time I entered medical school several years later, I had a solid footing in the science of nutrition. This allowed me to look at various disease processes and devise alternative nutritional therapies to augment or replace the traditional therapies. The beauty of nutritional therapies is that they treat the entire body and not just the symptoms. The result is a much healthier patient in all areas.

As I continued my research I discovered that one of the primary and most effective ways to control subclinical inflammation on a cellular level is through diet. You might wonder what this has to do with acne. The answer is everything! If we eat foods that generate a strong inflammatory response in the body, we are actually creating inflammation on a cellular level. This is important for many reasons. For starters, cellular inflammation accelerates the aging process, as well as the onset and natural course of many diseases—from cancer to cardiovascular disease, arthritis to acne. Although acne cannot be classified as a life-threatening disease, it is still extremely important to find ways to prevent and treat it.

Conversely, we can eat foods that are beneficial to the body because of their powerful anti-inflammatory properties. In the case of acne, the foods we eat are just as important as the foods we avoid. It is important to understand this basic concept. Once again, good old-fashioned common sense comes into play. The anti-inflammatory diet is based upon a well-balanced group of foods that we have been told since time immemorial

Here is but a small sample of the fantastic foods that not only taste great but do wonders for your skin (and help fight acne!)

Almonds	Honeydew melon
Apples	Kale
Artichokes	Kidney beans
Asparagus	Lentils
Barley	Macadamia nuts
Beans (dried and fresh)	Mushrooms
Bean sprouts	Oatmeal (regular, not
Berries (blackberries,	instant)
blueberries,	Oats
strawberries, etc.)	Olive oil
Bok choy	Olives
Brazil nuts	Oysters
Broccoli	Pears
Brussels sprouts	Pecans
Cabbage	Pinto beans
Cantaloupe	Pomegranate
Cauliflower	Pumpkin seeds
Celery	Red bell peppers
Cherries	Romaine lettuce
Chickpeas	Salmon
Chinese cabbage	Snow peas
Cucumbers	Soy products
Eggplant	Spinach
Endive	Sunflower seeds
Escarole	Tofu
Fish & Shellfish	Tomatoes
Flaxseed	Turkey
Green bell peppers	Turnips
Hazelnuts	Yogurt

are good for us. Most old adages have stood the test of time because they hold more than a glimmer of truth—from "fish is brain food" (one of the truest aphorisms every spoken) to "an apple a day keeps the doctor away."

The Sugar-Inflammation Connection

The key to the anti-inflammatory diet is that it has been designed to *prevent a rapid rise in blood sugar.* Why is this important? Because a rapid rise in blood sugar causes an insulin response in the body, which then causes an inflammatory response.[1] Remember this simple fact: whatever food we eat is converted to sugar as it is digested. Different foods are converted to sugar at varying rates. If we consume foods that are *rapidly* converted to sugar, that is considered proinflammatory. Proinflammatory foods cause all kinds of problems in the body resulting from a rapid rise in blood sugar, which in turn sparks a burst of inflammation on a cellular level. As our insulin rises, this triggers more inflammation throughout the body.[2]

Acne Alert! Inflammation-inducing Foods to Avoid

Bagels	Croissants
Bananas	Doughnuts
Breads, rolls	Dried fruits
Cake	Egg rolls
Candy	Flour
Cereals (except slow-cooking oatmeal)	French fries
	Fried food
Cookies	Fruit juices
Corn	Granola
Cornbread, corn muffins	Hard cheese (except
Cornstarch, Corn syrup	Romano and
Crackers	Parmesan)
Cream cheese	Honey

Hot dogs	Pizza
Ice cream, frozen yogurt,	Popcorn
Italian ice, sherbet	Potatoes
Jam, jelly, preserves	Pudding
Mango	Relish
Margarine	Rice
Molasses	Snack foods (e.g., potato
Muffins	chips, pretzels, corn
Noodles	chips, rice and corn
Pancakes	cakes, etc.)
Papaya	Soda
Pasta	Sugar (white and
Pastry	brown)
Peas	Tacos
Pie	Tortillas
Pita bread	Waffles

The cornerstone of the anti-inflammatory diet is the careful regulation of blood sugar. Never forget this important fact if you want to have clear, healthy, and beautiful skin. It is crucial to understand the relationship between the food we eat and its effect on blood sugar levels.

By now, almost everyone is aware that eating sweet foods such as cookies, cakes, and candy will cause a rise in blood sugar. Unfortunately, a lot of people are not aware that many foods not considered sweets are also rapidly converted to sugar in the body. In fact, at first glance many pro-inflammatory foods appear to be good choices. Just a few of these are bananas, potatoes, fruit juices, processed cereals, corn, peas, rice, pasta, bread—the list goes on. These simple starches are broken down into sugar by enzymes in the digestive system. Once these foods are ingested, they act the same as sweet foods, causing a rapid rise in blood sugar, triggering an increase in insulin, resulting in inflammation on a cellular level. (Elevated insulin levels also cause the body to store fat.)

Quality and Quantity—They Both Count

How can we tell which foods are proinflammatory, which foods are rapidly converted to sugar? As mentioned in the previous chapter, a rough index has been developed known as the glycemic index that rates food on an arbitrary scale from zero to one hundred. Water is zero and table sugar is one hundred. Foods with ratings above fifty should be avoided. The lower the rating on the glycemic index, the less likely it is to be proinflammatory. Proteins and fats, for example, rate low, while sugar and starchy foods rate high.

In addition to understanding the glycemic index, another important factor to consider is the *quantity*—the glycemic load—of the food eaten at a given time. If we eat too much at one sitting, even if the food is very low on the glycemic index, it will cause a rise in blood sugar. As always, common sense prevails: "Moderation in all things."

As you learn to control your blood sugar—which is the absolute key to controlling inflammation and thus preventing diseases, accelerated aging, cognitive impairment, and fatigue—it is important to be aware of the:

- *Types* of foods being eaten
- *Amount* of food being eaten *at any one time*

It is both the type of foods eaten and the amounts eaten that determine how rapidly blood sugar will rise. The key to the anti-inflammatory diet is learning how to carefully regulate blood sugar and insulin levels so that inflammation on a cellular level can be controlled. If one's blood sugar is high, inflammation runs rampant throughout the body, resulting in feeling (and looking) terrible, low energy levels, an increased susceptibility to infectious diseases, age-related diseases, and an accelerated aging process—as well as increased acne flare-ups. This proinflammatory state sets off a cascade of problems. The immune system is depressed, and levels of critical neurotransmitters are reduced, negatively affecting mood, cognitive abilities, and memory. An ongoing proinflammatory state slowly but surely destroys the body *and* the brain. To optimize health and keep skin clear and beautiful we must avoid proinflammatory foods, which include the aforementioned sugar and everything that is rapidly converted to sugar, such as potatoes, pasta, bread, sugar, honey, cakes, cookies, candy, baked goods, dried fruits, sugary beverages, sweet drinks of any kind.

But this is only half of the story. In addition to avoiding the pro-inflammatory foods, it is crucial to learn about the foods that have powerful *anti-inflammatory* activity. Many of these anti-inflammatory foods provide excellent sources of essential fatty acids (the good fats). The essential fatty acids designated as the omega 3s have powerful anti-inflammatory activity.[3] These good fats are found in many foods, including fish, salmon in particular. Fresh fruits and vegetables are also wonderful foods with anti-inflammatory properties.[4] Those possessing the most powerful anti-inflammatory activities are the ones that are brightest in color—Mother Nature's signal that they contain many antioxidants.[4,5] Antioxidants include vitamin C and vitamin E, as well as the carotenoids.

> **Remember this important fact:** all antioxidants act as anti-inflammatories. Foods that are rich in antioxidants are high in anti-inflammatory activity.[6,7]

I encourage everyone to drink at least eight to ten glasses of water every day. Taken in the proper quantities, water exerts an anti-inflammatory effect on our bodies, and when we combine plenty of water with the anti-inflammatory diet there is a very rapid reduction of inflammation in the body with visible results on the skin. To fight inflammation and get rid of acne, water is just as important as high-quality protein; essential fatty acids; and low-glycemic, antioxidant-rich carbohydrates. Believe it or not, I have seen dramatic improvement in patients' acne just by increasing their water intake.

The Three-Day Challenge

I have designed a simple, easy-to-follow three-day diet that changes the appearance of the skin so dramatically that its followers are often stopped by friends and colleagues who say, "You look different—what's your secret?" Their skin looks absolutely radiant and firm, dark under-eye circles disappear, and puffiness is reduced. This diet has been used time and time again as my preliminary anti-aging diet. The good news is that this three-day diet also works to rapidly improve the skin of acne sufferers.

I have included this three-day intensive anti-inflammatory diet at the end of this chapter so that you can jump-start your program for beautiful, healthy skin. Nothing motivates like success, and the three-day diet never fails—unless you cheat.

As you review the intensive three-day anti-inflammatory diet you will notice that it contains a lot of salmon (especially wild Alaskan salmon). Why is that? First of all, salmon is an excellent source of protein. We need good sources of protein to repair our cells, have a healthy immune system, and to fight off disease. In addition, salmon contains high levels of essential fatty acids such as the omega-3s. Omega-3s promote powerful anti-inflammatory activity, and when eaten with other nutritional foods, this anti-inflammatory effect can make a profound change in the course of acne as well as all the other diseases mentioned.

Salmon also contains a very important nutrient known as DMAE, which is short for a very long word: dimethylaminoethanol. In addition to being a natural anti-inflammatory, DMAE also helps improve nerve function. Having adequate amounts of DMAE in our diet can help improve thinking, problem-solving ability, and memory. In fact, DMAE was once used as a prescription medication for the treatment of attention deficit disorder and as a cognitive enhancer for conditions such as memory loss in adults. No wonder my grandma said that fish is brain food—its high levels of DMAE are responsible.

In addition to its function as a cognitive enhancer, DMAE is also a membrane stabilizer; that is, it protects the exterior of the cell. My years studying the causes of inflammation have convinced me that the cell plasma membrane is a source of many proinflammatory chemicals. This means that anything that stabilizes the outside of the cell plasma membrane acts as a natural anti-inflammatory.

Most cooking oils—such as corn, safflower, peanut, and soybean oils—are proinflammatory sources of omega-6 essential fatty acids, and tend to be over abundant in the average Western diet. However, omega-6s are essential when they are in the correct ratio to omega-3s. The preferred dietary ratio of omega-6 to omega-3 is two to one, but the omega-6 to omega-3 ratio of the average American diet is closer to thirty to one! I believe that the best source of omega-6 essential fatty acids is borage oil, because it provides an activated form of omega-6, a precursor of good prostaglandins, which assist cellular function. It is also very important to find good sources of omega-3s, such as fish, like wild Alaskan salmon,[8] and vegetarian sources such as flaxseed. Further, essential fatty acids can actually help stave off depression.[9] In fact, one small, but well-designed 1999 study by Harvard Medical School researchers showed that bipolar patients who had seen little relief from standard drugs improved markedly when given omega-3 essential fatty acid supplements. The researchers attributed this success to the ability of omega-3 fatty acids to stabilize the membrane of brain cells. Israeli researchers reported similar positive results in a 2002 follow-up study.[10]

I recommend incorporating extra virgin olive oil into the diet as much as possible. Although olive oil has low levels of essential fatty acids, it contains a fat called oleic acid, which actually helps the body absorb essential fatty acids more efficiently. Olive oil also contains a natural antioxidant called hydroxytyrosol, a polyphenol that has powerful anti-inflammatory activity.[11-13] It is no coincidence that in parts of the world, such as the Mediterranean, where olive oil is consumed in large amounts, people have a lower risk of heart disease, which is an inflammatory process. Toss out all other vegetable oils (other than cold-pressed flaxseed oil) and substitute extra virgin olive oil.

I also recommend that your daily diet contain lots of brightly colored fresh fruits and vegetables. When you're making a salad, use dark green lettuce like romaine as opposed to pale green, like iceberg. For dressings I recommend extra virgin olive oil mixed with the juice of a fresh lemon, to ensure plenty of antioxidants, which also function as powerful anti-inflammatories. For dessert, I recommend mixed berries—such as blueberries, raspberries, blackberries, and strawberries—and fresh melon, especially cantaloupe. Once again, notice the intense colors of these foods.

Bright color means there are lots of antioxidants present, which act as natural anti-inflammatories. Cantaloupe is also rich in vitamin A and has both hydrating and anti-inflammatory effects when eaten regularly.

As you look over the three-day diet, you will notice it is comprised of three small meals and two snacks evenly spaced throughout the day. This is to keep your blood sugar on an even keel and to ensure that your glycemic load stays at acceptable anti-inflammatory levels. Start each meal with a good source of protein, such as cold-water fish. Other good protein choices are chicken, turkey, soy products, and (occasionally) beef. Always eat your protein first, followed by a source of low-glycemic carbohydrates (such as bright-colored fruits and vegetables), and a source of high-quality essential fatty acids (such as chopped nuts or ground flaxseed added to your salad or yogurt; another good source is avocado). If you choose salmon, you are eating a combination of quality protein and essential fatty acids. As you sit down to each meal, check your plate to make sure that you have representatives from each of the critical three categories: protein, low-glycemic antioxidant carbohydrates, and essential fatty acids.

The initiation to the anti-inflammatory lifestyle by the three-day diet will clearly demonstrate to you that food does make a difference. When you look in the mirror at the end of the three days you will find a major incentive to continue with my 28-Day Program—a must if your goal is acne-free skin. The three-day diet is not as diverse as the 28-Day Program—but an intense program is necessary to see visible results in just three days. The good news? Once you finish the three day diet and see the difference, you can move on to the 28-Day Program, which includes a broader choice of foods, ensuring that you will never feel denied or bored.

This is not a low-calorie or low-fat diet. Neither is the solution to clear skin—or weight control for that matter. Salmon, olive oil, nuts, and avocados all contain fats. But they are the healthy, skin-clearing, skin-beautifying fats—and they will not make you fat. Another myth foisted upon us by the scientific community is that fat is dangerous and should be avoided at all cost. Thanks to high-carbohydrate, low-fat, no-fat diets slavishly followed over the past fifteen years or so, this country is now plagued by an epidemic of obesity, serious mental depression (the brain is dependent upon essential fatty acids to function correctly), depressed immune systems, wrinkled and/or acne-prone skin, and an increased risk of stroke, heart disease, and diabetes. Learn to recognize the goods fats such as I have outlined in my program.

Equally important is to avoid bad fats, especially the trans fats common in baked goods, French fries, chips, cookies, crackers, and snack foods—all foods that are highly proinflammatory. Trans fats are not natural; they are man-made and are found in food products whose labels contain the words "partially hydrogenated." In addition to baked and fried foods, many convenience foods contain trans fats, as do popular brands of peanut butter and shortening. You should avoid these scrupulously. When you follow the anti-inflammatory diet—which is rich in vitamins, antioxidants, essential fatty acids, and protein—you will be carefully controlling your blood sugar and insulin levels, decreasing inflammation in your body, and decreasing your risk for every age-related disease, including the disease of aging. Your skin will be clear and beautiful; and when your skin is beautiful on the outside, you know that you are doing well on the inside. Remember, beauty comes from the inside and the skin is the perfect reflection of what is going on inside of your body.

Now, let's take a look at the effects of the average American high-glycemic diet on the onset and course of acne. As we have learned, acne is an inflammatory disease that develops in stages.[14] The early stages are characterized by the interior of the pores getting clogged with skin cells that have been shed yet not removed. This is known as *retention hyperkeratosis*. A proinflammatory diet creates retention hyperkeratosis by several mechanisms:[15]

- An increase in blood sugar causes the release of proinflammatory cytokines such as IL-1, causing retention hyperkeratosis (sticky cells in the follicle).
- Rapid increase in blood sugar causes changes in the endocrine system, including the release of growth hormone and insulin, which can cause increased proliferation of cells in the follicle.
- Increased inflammation on a cellular level caused by diet can alter energy production in the sebaceous gland resulting in increased sebum production.

- Changes in energy production in the sebaceous gland result in an abnormal ratio of proinflammatory fatty acids.
- Abnormal production of fatty acids can mimic molecules similar to a platelet-activating factor, which act as messengers to the body to produce inflammation.

Also, retention hyperkeratosis can result in the stretching of the follicular wall, resulting in disruption of the cell plasma membrane. This prompts a release of phospholipids, which are then broken down into proinflammatory chemicals. Human toll-like receptors found on certain cells result in the production of inflammatory cytokines; these toll-like receptor positive cells are abundant around the so-called noninflammatory acne lesions.

Once the pores clog, the oils and bacteria build up, forming the primary lesion known as the comedo. Once again, this is the term physicians use for a clogged pore. Physicians categorize this type of early lesion as a noninflamed acne lesion. Once again, they are wrong. Why do they call it noninflamed acne? Well, when they look under the microscope, they don't see signs of inflammation. But the fact is, inflammation begins here, in the very first lesion—in fact, it had begun before that first lesion even formed. In addition cytokines are being secreted in the lesions. These cytokines, or cellular messengers, are evident even before retention hyperkeratosis takes place.[16,17] Transcription factors such as NF-kappa B activate cytokines, which signal the cell to produce even more inflammatory chemicals.

Research is currently being conducted into the presence of cytokines and transcription factors in acne. But this research is looking at their presence in only what is considered the inflammatory lesions of acne. Researchers have still failed to focus on the preventative aspect of treating early so-called noninflamed, or Grade 1 lesions with anti-inflammatory therapy. Physicians need to understand that proinflammatory cytokines exist in the pore even before *Propionibacterium acnes* bacteria is present. I take comfort in knowing that the research into cytokine activity in inflammatory lesions will advance knowledge to the point that physicians may someday understand the effects of cytokines on these so-called noninflammatory lesions.

I find it hard to grasp that in this day and age, when every physician and scientist knows that there are molecules that indicate inflammation, and molecules that are far too small to be seen by a microscope, the prevailing conclusion is that noninflamed acne lesions exist. Be that as it may, the so-called noninflamed acne lesion (which certainly is inflamed, regardless of what conventional wisdom posits) is the closed comedo, commonly known as a whitehead. This type of early lesion is also characterized as Grade One acne, or the mildest form of acne. The next lesion categorized by doctors is the open comedo, or blackhead. These lesions appear to be black because the oils inside the clogged pore have oxidized. They also contain melanin, the pigment found in our skin.

The Power of the Anti-inflammatory Diet in Stopping Acne

Here is where we can directly interfere with the formation of acne lesions. By following an anti-inflammatory diet, we can actually reduce the level of cytokines in the proinflammatory fatty acids that are secreted by the sebaceous cell, thus avoiding the onset of new acne lesions and radically altering the course of existing acne. In addition, by following an anti-inflammatory diet, we can prevent the inflammatory consequences of acne, such as scarring, which may be irreversible—particularly in adult acne sufferers.

The Three-Day Skin-Clear Jump-Start Program

The daily menus on this three-day diet are very similar. Though there is some variety, my patients have told me that the program is easier to follow when choices are limited. Don't worry: the foods are delicious and healthful, and you will be very pleased with the fast, impossible-to-ignore results.

Planning is everything. Be sure to pick a three-day period during which it will be easy to control what you eat (for example, not during holiday or vacation). Go to the grocery store and stock up on the ingredi-

Helpful Skin-Clearing Jump-Start Tips

· Flaxseed can be purchased in your local health food store. Keep it in your freezer and grind small amounts as needed in a food mill. Sprinkle ground flaxseed liberally on your oatmeal, yogurt, salads. Your skin will thank you for making the effort!

· No coffee, juice, bread. Eat only what is on the menu.

· Always eat protein first!

· Drink at least eight 8-ounce glasses of pure spring water each day. If desired, squeeze a fresh lemon into your water or garnish with fresh lemon slices.

· Keep bottles of water in convenient spots so it is always close at hand.

ents you'll need for the three-day diet before you begin. Buy the freshest foods you can find, and get rid of the bad foods you might have on hand that may tempt you to stray.

WAKE UP
- 8 ounces spring water

BREAKFAST
- 2 egg omelet or a 4- to 6-ounce piece of grilled or broiled salmon
- ½ cup cooked oatmeal (not instant) topped with 1 tablespoon ground flaxseed
- 3-inch slice cantaloupe or ¼ cup fresh berries (blueberries are especially good).
- 8 ounces spring water
- Green or black tea

LUNCH
- 4 to 6 ounces grilled salmon *or* sardines packed in olive oil (see resource section)

- 2 cups romaine lettuce; dress with extra virgin olive oil and freshly squeezed lemon juice to taste
- 2-inch slice cantaloupe and ¼ cup fresh berries
- 8 ounces spring water

MID-AFTERNOON SNACK
- Apple
- 6 ounces plain yogurt
- ¼ cup pumpkin seeds
- 8 ounces spring water (minimum, more if desired)

DINNER
- 4 to 6 ounces grilled salmon
- 2 cups romaine lettuce; dress with extra virgin olive oil and freshly squeezed lemon juice to taste
- ½ cup steamed vegetables (especially bright green vegetables, such as asparagus, broccoli, spinach)
- 2-inch slice cantaloupe
- 8 ounces spring water

BEFORE-BEDTIME SNACK
- 2 ounces sliced turkey breast
- ¼ cup blueberries
- 3 or 4 pecans or almonds
- 8 ounces spring water

And there you have it! What could be easier? If you've stuck to this diet, after three days you should see the results—clearer skin: diminished blemishes, decreased redness—in your mirror. And if, as I suspect, you now know that what you eat does have a very real effect on your acne, read on and learn all about acne and my three-tiered approach (diet, supplements, and topicals) to its treatment.

5

The Three-Tiered Perricone
Anti-Acne Program—
Tier 2: Nutritional Supplements

As I mentioned in Chapter Four, before I entered medical school, I was fortunate enough to spend many years studying nutrition and the effects of nutritional supplements on health. I learned that nutritional supplements—such as vitamins, minerals, and other nutrients, as well as amino acids—have profound effects on health and the treatment of disease. This background knowledge exerted a major influence on me during my years in medical school. It was the reason that I looked for a nutritional and/or nutritional supplement solution whenever I approached any disease process. With every case, I asked myself the following question: "How can a change in diet or nutritional supplementation affect the clinical course of this patient's disease?"

While today this might seem a normal and necessary line of inquiry for the enlightened physician to pursue, when I was in school this was not the case. Medical schools did not teach nutrition in any formal manner at all! In fact, I soon learned that there was an obvious bias *against* nutritional supplements—not only on the part of the curriculum writers and my immediate professors but also within the greater medical community.

However, as readers of *The Perricone Prescription* and *The Wrinkle Cure* know, I was not about to let a little bias stop me. This would not be the first or last time I challenged the status quo during the course of my medical education. Consequently I found myself embroiled in some rather interesting and spirited discussions with my professors when I suggested the employment of certain nutritional supplements in the treatment of various disease processes. The resistance and often downright hostility accorded my theories made me realize that I was not going to turn the medical profession around during my medical training. I remained undaunted. After all, I was living proof of the turnaround that can be achieved by means of changes in diet and the addition of targeted nutritional supplements. Still, I couldn't help but be amazed at the prevailing archaic attitude. Here I was, in the midst of securing the finest medical education available, and something so intrinsic to our physical and mental condition—the food we eat—was considered to play *no* role in sickness or in health.

From the chapters you have already read, you have learned that acne is a systemic inflammatory disease with many contributing factors. These factors are diverse, and they consist of metabolic and energy-producing changes, hormonal influences, oil gland activity, and genetic predisposition. We must always remember that despite all the contributing factors, the final common pathway is inflammation. By understanding the biochemistry underlying the cellular processes, we can control acne.

Vitamin A

A simple case in point is to look at vitamin A and acne. In other chapters we have discussed the importance of vitamin A derivatives for the treatment of acne. Now I want to demonstrate how vitamin A can fit into the larger picture. Vitamin A is used in systemic treatments in drugs such as Accutane; it is also used in topical treatments using vitamin A derivatives such as Retin A or vitamin A acid.

Why was the discovery of the efficacy of vitamin A derivatives such a breakthrough? Because it is a perfect example of the far-reaching powers of nutritional supplements, when they are properly applied.

My three-tiered approach to health can be used to illustrate this because vitamin A and (many other important supplements) have dietary components, a nutritional supplement component, and a topical component—and they all work synergistically when correctly integrated into a program.

Vitamin A, which is found in many foods, controls the development of epithelial cells, which are a component of skin that lines all the mucosal membranes in the body. Vitamin A is important in the process of keratinization, in which the epidermis migrates and matures into the stratum corneum. And yet it is the derivatives of vitamin A that are important in treating acne, and *not* the natural form of vitamin A.

Why is natural vitamin A not considered therapeutic? The answer lies in the fact that natural vitamin A is responsible for maintaining the normal maturation of the skin. However, to treat abnormal processes such as acne, large doses must be given, which then results in vitamin A toxicity. Vitamin A acid—also known as Retin-A, tretinoin, or retinoic acid—is a derivative form of Retin-A that is active in skin. Water-soluble derivatives of vitamin A, such as Accutane, may therefore be given systemically in very high doses without the toxicity resulting from large doses of natural vitamin A. However, Accutane has significant side effects, as discussed in Chapter Two, making it imperative that patients undergoing a course of Accutane be under a physician's care.

Zinc

One of the few nutritional supplements that dermatologists consider to be therapeutic in treating acne is zinc. Zinc is a mineral that is essential to all aspects of our health. Zinc is found in more than two hundred enzymes that are important to our cellular health. Zinc is important for the function of transcription factors, as it allows them to interact with the DNA in the cell nuclei. Zinc is vital for our bodies' growth and development and is essential in sex and reproduction. Zinc deficiency can cause severe growth problems, and it is critical to the proper functioning of the immune system. Zinc has some antioxidant activity, as well as a powerful anti-inflammatory activity. Several studies in which patients were given zinc supplement capsules resulted in improvement of acne. Some physicians recommend up to 100 milligrams of zinc supplements a day for the treatment of acne. However, these higher doses may result in nausea, vomiting, and stomach pain. Pregnant women and nursing mothers should not take zinc in doses higher than 15 milligrams per day to avoid causing harm to the fetus or child. As always, I strongly recommend that you consult your primary physician if you are pregnant or nursing before undertaking any dietary, supplement, or exercise program.

Alpha Lipoic Acid

Alpha lipoic acid is a powerful nutritional substance that has both antioxidant and anti-inflammatory activity. Alpha lipoic acid is found naturally in our bodies in the tiny energy-producing portion of the cell known as the *mitochondriona,* which is responsible for the conversion of food to energy. Alpha lipoic acid has been called the metabolic antioxidant because it aids in the production of energy from food.

Alpha lipoic acid is part of an enzyme complex known as *pyruvate dehydrogenase,* which is essential in energy conversion. Within our cells, alpha lipoic acid is locked in this enzyme complex and does not move freely about the cells. We cannot get enough alpha lipoic acid from our diet, as only small amounts of it are found in food. Fortunately, in 1951 scientists were able to identify the structure of alpha lipoic acid, resulting in the synthesis of this amazing substance. This means that alpha lipoic acid can now be taken orally in supplement form and/or applied topically directly onto the skin, where it can move freely within the cell delivering its maximum benefits to all parts of the cell.

When alpha lipoic acid is free in the cell, it has a powerful antioxidant activity that has been described by some scientists as having four hundred times the antioxidant activity of vitamins C and E combined. One of the chief benefits that comes from taking alpha lipoic acid supplements is a feeling of increased energy. An added bonus is that many patients report a decrease in body fat when they take this powerful antioxidant. Alpha lipoic acid is a unique antioxidant because it is both fat and water soluble. Many antioxidants, such as vitamin C in the form of ascorbic acid, are water soluble, meaning that they only reach the watery portions of the cell, while leaving the parts of the cell composed of fats unprotected. Other antioxidants, such as vitamin E, are fat soluble, reaching only the fat-soluble portions of the cells. As alpha lipoic acid is both fat and water soluble, it has earned the title of universal antioxidant—it can reach all portions of the cell, providing superior protection from free-radical damage and inflammation.

The Acne Connection

Alpha lipoic acid is extremely valuable in the treatment of acne because it helps control both blood sugar and insulin. As we have discussed before, a rapid rise in blood sugar may produce a burst of inflammation that elevates insulin levels, which then affect many other hormones in our endocrine system. This results in the formation of new acne lesions, as well as exacerbating any existing acne. When we are able to stabilize blood sugar levels we can also better control insulin levels. Alpha lipoic acid can control blood sugar by both sensitizing the cell to the effects of insulin and allowing the cell to better utilize blood sugar.

Alpha lipoic acid exerts powerful anti-inflammatory effects through several mechanisms of action.[1-4] First of all, it protects the cell plasma membrane. Alpha lipoic acid prevents this membrane from breaking down into proinflammatory chemicals (such as arachidonic acid), which can then flow into the cell, causing damage. Arachidonic acid is broken down into prostaglandins and other proinflammatory chemicals that can affect cellular integrity. Alpha lipoic acid protects the cell plasma membrane from free radical damage, which activates these destructive proinflammatory chemicals. In addition, alpha lipoic acid can act on the cytosol (the internal portion of the cell) by preventing the production of the proinflammatory cytokines.

Transcription Factors and Gene Expression

Our cellular processes, including gene expression, are controlled by various proteins within the cell. Transcription factors are tiny proteins whose job is to carry messages to the nucleus, or the DNA. NfkB is an important transcription factor in cell inflammation. NfkB is a protein that remains in the inner portion of the cell and is completely inactive unless the cell experiences an increase in free radicals or the cell experiences an increase in inflammatory chemicals. Either will result in oxidative stress. Under these conditions, a small inhibitory portion of the transcription factor NfkB is cleaved off, allowing the NfkB to reach the nucleus of the cell, activating DNA. This results in the production of proinflammatory cytokines, such as tumor necrosis factor alpha and interleukins, as I discuss in my previous books. Levels of these proinflammatory cytokines are then elevated in the cell, generating free radicals and causing further damage to the cell.

Alpha Lipoic Acid to the Rescue

Alpha lipoic acid inhibits the activation of NfkB, thereby suppressing the inflammatory response within the cell. This means that alpha lipoic acid is a powerful tool against the inflammation that is seen in acne. In addition, alpha lipoic acid also controls another transcription factor called AP-1 which is activated when a cell is under oxidative stress—that is, when there is an excess of free radicals and not enough protection from antioxidants. Once activated, AP-1 heads straight for the nucleus of the cell where it activates genes that control the production of enzymes that can digest collagen. This digestion of collagen is actually one of the causative factors in the birth of a wrinkle. However, AP-1 has another—and just as important—corollary for the acne patient: An inflammatory acne lesion results in the activation of transcription factor AP-1 which then produces enzymes that digest the surrounding collagen. The result is scarring.

By suppressing inflammation on a cellular level, alpha lipoic acid can help prevent scarring from active acne lesions.[5,6] This is very good news because about the only thing worse than an unsightly acne lesion is a lifetime reminder of it in the form of a deep scar or pockmark. It is also important to note that alpha lipoic acid exerts an even greater action on AP-1. AP-1 is not only activated by the destructive free radicals but also it can be activated by alpha lipoic acid! On the face of it, this does not sound like good news. However, there is a significant difference in the effects. When AP-1 is activated by alpha lipoic acid, the enzymes activated by

AP-1 digest only *damaged* collagen. Because scars are made up of damaged collagen, alpha lipoic acid can actually reverse existing scar tissue. This fact alone makes alpha lipoic acid a miracle worker in fighting acne and repairing the damage left by this disfiguring disease. In Chapter Six, we will examine in greater detail just how this and other topical formulations of superstar anti-inflammatories, such as DMAE, can dramatically reduce scars associated with acne and other problems. I recommend taking between 50 to 100 milligrams per day of alpha lipoic acid as a dietary supplement. Unless advised by your physician, do not take alpha lipoic acid while you are pregnant.

Pantothenic Acid (Vitamin B$_5$)

Pantothenic acid is an amazing nutrient. It is part of a molecule known as coenzyme A, which is essential for energy production in the body. Pantothenic acid is concentrated in the adrenal glands where it is necessary for the production of hormones, including the stress hormone cortisol. In addition, pantothenic acid is essential for both the production and the stabilization of the sex hormones. Pantothenic acid is a key nutrient in some of our most important biochemical reactions.

With what we have learned about the sex hormones, such as testosterone, and the stress hormones, such as cortisol, and the roles they play in acne, it is easy to see how this essential nutrient might be of great benefit. It should also be noted that pantothenic acid is important in the production and utilization of fats in our body—again, a key area of interest and concern for the acne patient. Even a small deficiency of pantothenic acid will result in the abnormal utilization of fats and fatty acids. When we are under stress and thus producing excess cortisol, the pantothenic acid in our bodies is rapidly metabolized and used up. This results in lower amounts of pantothenic acid available for the proper utilization of fats and for maintaining the proper ratio of sex steroids in the body. Thus, it makes sense that when we are under stress, acne flares up. Lack of pantothenic acid also contributes to a rise in blood sugar, bringing on a burst of inflammation as a result of the body's decreased ability to properly utilize fatty acids.[7] This in turn leads to abnormal secretions in the sebaceous gland, which, we know, is a hallmark of acne.

In several studies, pantothenic acid supplements have significantly improved the course of acne for many patients. Pantothenic acid is extremely nontoxic and the dosages can vary greatly, anywhere from 10 milligrams all the way up to several thousand milligrams a day. Other benefits of pantothenic acid include its powerful antioxidant and anti-inflammatory activity—two qualities I look for when searching for therapies for everything from acne to aging. Finally, pantothenic acid also protects the cell plasma membrane from lipid peroxidation, which is a condition that results in the oxidation of important fats in the cell. Again, pantothenic acid is extremely non-toxic and I am not aware of any reports of a pantothenic acid over-dosage. However, pregnant women and nursing mothers should avoid taking more than 10 milligrams per day without the explicit direction of their physicians.

DMAE (dimethylaminoethanol)

DMAE, or dimethylaminoethanol, a nutritional substance with powerful anti-inflammatory properties, is found in high levels in fish such as salmon—especially wild Alaskan salmon. DMAE works by stabilizing the outer layer of the cell known as the cell plasma membrane. In addition to its anti-inflammatory activities, DMAE is important in the production of neurotransmitters, chemicals that affect the nerves. DMAE is a building block of the neurotransmitter acetylcholine, which plays an important role in the communication between brain cells and other nerve cells. Acetylcholine is essential in the communication of one nerve to another and also in the communication between nerves and muscles. In order for your muscles to contract, the message has to be sent from your nerves to your muscles via acetylcholine.

Because DMAE is a building block for acetylcholine, taking it as a supplement at therapeutic levels has been shown to increase cognitive function, that is, improve memory and problem-solving ability. It has also been shown to affect improvement in such conditions as attention deficit disorder (ADD). DMAE can also affect muscle tone, as muscle tone can be increased when additional acetylcholine is provided. This is very exciting because it gives us a way to actually improve our appearance by counteracting the sagging associated with aging and acne scarring.

Because DMAE has powerful anti-inflammatory activity, it can also affect the transcription factor AP-1, resulting in diminished appearance of acne scars. A landmark study in which DMAE and alpha lipoic acid were combined in a topical solution showed marked resolution in scarring for patients with surgical scars, when applied twice daily. And, in a clinical trial of topical DMAE and alpha lipoic acid conducted in my own practice, fifteen patients showed an 80 percent reduction in the severity of their atrophic (indented) acne scars.[8] DMAE can be taken in supplemental doses of 50 to 100 milligrams per day. As always, pregnant and nursing women must consult their physician before taking this or any supplement.

Essential Fatty Acids

As my readers know by now, I am huge fan of essential fatty acids (EFAs). The omega-3 and omega-6 essential fatty acids are just that—essential fats necessary for the performance of many biochemical processes in the body. We know that omega-3s have powerful anti-inflammatory activity.[9] Ensuring that we are getting enough essential fatty acids in our diet is one of the best ways we have to help fight the systemic anti-inflammatory disease of acne.

What exactly are essential fatty acids and what role do they play in treating and preventing acne? The following material is adapted from *The Perricone Prescription,* as it provides much that is relevant to the treatment of acne.

Fat is one of the nutrients your body requires, along with proteins, carbohydrates, and vitamins. The building blocks of fats and oils are called fatty acids. The essential fatty acids are those fats that we can't make in our body. We must obtain them from our food.

The essential fatty acids, like omega-3s, are famous for their heart-protective effects. They can lower blood pressure, decrease the chance of blood clots, and offer a wide range of health benefits. Studies have shown that even small amounts of fish in the diet can lower risk of colon, breast, and prostate cancers. Doctors have found that the pain and inflammation of severe rheumatoid arthritis (another autoimmune disease on the rise and targeting women) is reduced by omega-3s.[10] Laboratory studies of psoriasis patients indicate that they are low in omega-3. When treated with fish oil concentrates high in omega-3s, these patients find that their itchy, scaly patches improve. The omega-3 essential fatty acids dramatically reduce the body's production of inflammatory compounds.[10] They actually block the production of arachidonic acid, a major cause of inflammation in the body. Omega-3 fatty acids are particularly good at targeting leukotrienes, chemicals that are provoked by the presence of free radicals and are known to promote allergies and skin disorders.

Two omega-3 oils, EPA and DHA, are found in high levels in salmon. It was once thought that most of fish's positive effects on the cardiovascular system were due to its EPA content of the essential fatty acids. We have since discovered that the DHA portion is also very important to cardiovascular health. DHA is seen to be more powerful in lowering triglycerides and increasing levels of the good cholesterol, HDL. At the same time, DHA also has a marked effect in lowering blood pressure. But omega-3s are not the only EPAs that have been shown to be beneficial to cardiovascular health.

The omega-6 oils are also extremely beneficial. Their active ingredients are derived from linoleic acid. Pumpkin seed oil is 45 percent linoleic acid. Linoleic acid has widespread effects throughout the body due to its effect on membrane function. Acne patients have a low concentration of linoleic acid in their sebum, and the levels decrease as the severity of acne increases.[11,12] Supplementation with oils high in linoleic acid appears to improve the clinical course of patients on low-fat diets,* whatever the reason.[13] Of course, if you follow the Perricone Prescription for acne, you know it is important to avoid a low-fat diet. Eat plenty of pumpkin seeds and nuts in their natural states—unsalted and un-

---

* Downing, D.T., et al. "Essential Fatty Acids and Acne Vulgaris," *Journal of the American Academy of Dermatology* 14 (1986): pp. 221–25.

roasted—to ensure that your body has the skin-clearing essential fatty acids it needs to stay acne free.

Linoleic Acid

GLA, one derivative of the omega-6 parent molecule, linoleic acid, has also been shown to have a positive effect on lowering cholesterol and triglyceride levels by increasing the good cholesterol, HDL. Borage oil is the richest source of GLA, a metabolic product of linoleic acid that plays an important role in metabolic processes that positively influence premenstrual syndrome, menopause, obesity, and acne.

Both omega-6 and omega-3 help lower levels of stress chemicals. Norepinephrine is a chemical that is elevated in the blood during long-term stress. DHA significantly reduces norepinephrine levels in people who are chronically stressed. As they age, many people become overweight and experience increased stress, which makes their cells resistant to the effect of insulin. Their insulin levels continue to rise, but their blood sugar is not lowered. This state is known as insulin resistance, a condition that often occurs in people who have elevated levels of blood fats and heart disease and in type 2 diabetes. Research overwhelmingly indicates that GLA and DHA improve cell sensitivity to insulin, and thus reduce the chances of developing heart disease, diabetes, excess body fat, and acne.[14-16]

Brain function is intimately tied to our essential fatty acid intake. Remember, essential fatty acids make up the phospholipid bilayer of the cell membrane. This is critical to our brains' nerve cells. There are high levels of DHA in human milk, and children who are nursed have optimal brain growth and development as infants. Deficiencies of DHA can lead to such problems as attention deficit hyperactivity disorder, which has become epidemic in this country; increased aggression; and a higher incidence of Alzheimer's disease later in life.

Essential fatty acids work via an extremely powerful mechanism on a cellular level. Essential fatty acids affect transcription factors (tiny protein messengers) that then go to the nucleus of the cell, where directions are given by the nucleus that regulate fatty acid metabolism. The transcription factors affected by essential fatty acids are called *PPARs,* which stands for perixosome proliferator-activated receptors.[17] The receptors activate certain portions of the DNA that in turn affect all fatty acids on a cellular level. GLA and DHA activate PPARs and therefore affect gene transcription. Gene transcription is the activation of genes that results in control of all functions of the cell.

When your diet does not include sufficient amounts of essential fatty acids, wounds cannot heal and you are more susceptible to infections. Your face and body become dehydrated—and you know what that does to your looks! Lack of essential fatty acids can cause sterility in men, miscarriages in women, arthritis-like problems, and some heart and circulatory problems.

The Perricone Prescription List of Recommended Supplements

In addition to the nutrients mentioned above, it is important to include the following supplements to maintain optimum skin and body health. The following listing of recommended supplements (reprinted from my book *The Perricone Prescription*) has been designed for quick and easy reference for all of the nutrients we need. You will find listed for each nutrient:

- The features and benefits
- The symptoms and effects of a deficiency
- The best noninflammatory food sources
- The reference daily intake (RDI). In most cases, the RDI doses are identical to the U.S. RDA doses. (We use RDI here since federal law requires manufacturers to express the amount of nutrients in their products in terms of the percent of the RDI. The RDIs are the minimum doses needed to prevent nutrient-deficiency symptoms. I generally recommend doses of vitamins and minerals somewhat higher than the RDI levels.
- The no observed adverse effects level (NOAEL): the maximum daily dose that does not produce adverse effects, according to the Council for Responsible Nutrition. Certain nutrients are safe and

more supportive of optimal health at even higher doses (for example, high-dose niacin for improving blood cholesterol levels)—levels that may, in some circumstances, produce noninjurious adverse effects. The NOAEL doses are the maximums I would ever recommend. Pregnant or lactating women should not exceed the RDI except under a doctor's direction.

• The Acne-Free recommendation: the daily dose the average healthy adult should take to receive the maximum health and cosmetic benefits each supplement can provide. Check with your physician to be sure that these doses are appropriate for your individual health status and will not interact negatively with any drugs you take.

(See Resources for a list of companies from which you can order the vitamins for the program.)

Starting with the ABCs

Vitamins are either fat soluble or water soluble. Vitamins A, D, E, and K are fat soluble. They are stored in the liver and used up by the body very slowly. A buildup of these fat-soluble vitamins can be toxic. The B-complex vitamins and vitamin C are water soluble. The body uses these vitamins very quickly, and excess amounts are eliminated in urine. Vitamin A, the B-complex vitamins, and vitamin C are the foundation of my nutritional antiaging and anti-acne regimens.

Vitamin A
FEATURES AND BENEFITS
• Fat soluble
• Essential for growth
• Aids bone development
• Strengthens immune system
• Improves night vision
• Helps reproduction

- Promotes wound healing
- Encourages healthy skin

SYMPTOMS AND EFFECTS OF A VITAMIN A DEFICIENCY
- Disorder of the eye and epithelial tissues (the skin and mucous membranes lining the internal body surfaces)
- Rough, dry skin

NONINFLAMMATORY FOOD SOURCES
- Broccoli
- Cantaloupe
- Cod
- Halibut
- Kale
- Red bell peppers
- Spinach
- Watercress

INTAKE REQUIREMENTS AND SUPPLEMENT RECOMMENDATIONS
- RDI: 5,000 IU
- No observed adverse effects level: 10,000 IU
- Acne-Free recommendation: 5,000 to 10,000 IU from carotinoid sources

Vitamin A is part of a group of compounds called retinoids. It is found in animal products like liver, dairy products, eggs, and fish liver oil; it is also found in dark-red, green, and yellow vegetables. Vitamin A is best absorbed in the presence of some dietary fat and with sufficient zinc,

> The most popular prescription for acne and aging skin is topical Retin-A, an acid form of vitamin A. Retinol, the alcohol form of vitamin A, is used in cosmetics because it is converted in the skin into small amounts of Retin-A.

vitamin E, and protein in the body. As with all fat-soluble vitamins, excessive intake of vitamin A is toxic—unless you take it in the form of carotenes that the body converts to vitamin A on an as-needed basis.

Vitamin A helps cells reproduce normally, in a process known as differentiation. Cells that have not properly differentiated are more likely to undergo precancerous changes. Vitamin A is important for the health and integrity of the cell plasma membrane. As a fat-soluble antioxidant, it can get into the cell, provide protection, neutralize free radicals, and prevent oxidative stress.

A half-cup serving of broccoli, spinach, or cantaloupe contains enough vitamin A (in its precursor form, carotene) to meet the RDA for this nutrient. For antioxidant benefits, I recommend between 5,000 and 10,000 IU of vitamin A each day. Bear in mind that the liver stores vitamin A—and a buildup can be toxic. To avoid problems, do not exceed dosage recommendations for this and other fat-soluble vitamins. It is also important to note that many foods that are high in vitamin A can cause an inflammatory response as a result of their high sugar content. These include sweet potatoes, carrots, and yams, which I recommend that you avoid.

Vitamin B Complex
FEATURES AND BENEFITS
- Increased health of skin, hair, and nails
- Strengthens bones and muscles
- Improves energy production
- Helps metabolic function
- Aids protein digestion
- Promotes nervous system health
- Fortifies mucosal membranes
- Stimulates healthy intestinal and bowel function
- Prevents moodiness, restlessness, irritability, insomnia, and fatigue
- Improves liver health
- Reinforces proper brain cell function
- Prevents skin disorders
- Relieves PMS

SYMPTOMS AND EFFECTS OF A VITAMIN B COMPLEX DEFICIENCY
- Many skin disorders
- Nervousness
- Depression
- Lethargy
- Forgetfulness
- Insomnia

There are eight B vitamins in the Perricone supplement program:

- Vitamin B_1 (thiamin)
- Vitamin B_2 (riboflavin)
- Vitamin B_3 (niacin)
- Vitamin B_5 (pantothenic acid)
- Vitamin B_6 (pyridoxine)
- Vitamin B_{12} (cyanocobalamin)
- Folic acid (folate)
- Biotin

Most of the B vitamins are recognized as coenzymes that, taken together, work synergistically to perform essential biological processes—especially those affecting the nerves, brain, and skin.

This group of vitamins is water soluble, which means that they are not stored in the body and must be replenished each day. Let's take a closer look at each of the B vitamins.

Vitamin B_1 (Thiamin)
FEATURES AND BENEFITS
- Stimulates conversion of carbohydrates and glucose into energy
- Helps metabolism of proteins and fats
- Promotes healthy growth in childhood and adolescence
- Aids digestion
- Improves mental attitude
- Promotes normal function of the nervous system, muscles, and heart

SYMPTOMS AND EFFECTS OF A VITAMIN B_1 DEFICIENCY

- Problems with gastrointestinal, cardiovascular, and peripheral nervous systems
- Depression
- Irritability
- Attention deficit
- Muscular weakness

NONINFLAMMATORY FOOD SOURCES

- Chickpeas
- Pinto beans
- Raw nuts
- Salmon
- Soybeans

INTAKE REQUIREMENTS AND SUPPLEMENT RECOMMENDATIONS

- RDI: 1.5 mg
- No observed adverse effects level: 50 mg
- Acne-Free recommendation: 10 to 50 mg

Vitamin B_2 (Riboflavin)

FEATURES AND BENEFITS

- Essential for normal cell growth
- Helps metabolize carbohydrates, fats, and proteins
- Promotes healthy skin, hair, and nails

SYMPTOMS AND EFFECTS OF A VITAMIN B_2 DEFICIENCY

- Sores and cracks at the corners of the mouth
- Inflammation of the tongue and skin

NONINFLAMMATORY FOOD SOURCES

- Almonds
- Cottage cheese
- Milk
- Walnuts
- Yogurt

INTAKE REQUIREMENTS AND SUPPLEMENT RECOMMENDATIONS
- RDI: 1.7 mg
- No observed adverse effects level: 200 mg
- Acne-Free recommendation: 10 to 100 mg

Vitamin B$_3$ (Niacin)

FEATURES AND BENEFITS
- Aids cellular and lipid metabolism
- Maintains healthy skin
- Helps synthesize hormones
- Supports gastrointestinal and nervous system health
- Protects against carcinogens, preventing certain types of cancer
- Reduces cholesterol and triglyceride levels
- Treats and prevents circulatory problems
- Maintains mental stability

SYMPTOMS AND EFFECTS OF A VITAMIN B$_3$ DEFICIENCY
- Dermatitis (an inflammatory skin condition)
- Diarrhea
- Dementia
- Eye redness
- Loss of appetite
- Anxiety or nervousness

NONINFLAMMATORY FOOD SOURCES
- Almonds
- Hazelnuts
- Sunflower seeds
- Yogurt

INTAKE REQUIREMENTS AND SUPPLEMENT RECOMMENDATIONS
- RDI: 20 mg.
- No observed adverse effects level: 500 mg (Note: Doses of 1,000 to 4,000 mg a day are used for cholesterol control and, while generally safe, may produce side effects such as hot flushes, nausea,

and heartburn. Never take more than 500 mg a day of niacin without medical supervision.)
- Acne-Free recommendation: 20 to 100 mg

Vitamin B$_5$ (Pantothenic Acid)

FEATURES AND BENEFITS
- Promotes Krebs cycle of energy production (takes place in the mitochondria)
- Helps production of adrenal hormones
- Reduces cholesterol and triglyceride levels
- Plays a role in metabolism of fats, carbohydrates, and proteins
- Helps fight infection
- Increases physical endurance
- Improves body's ability to heal
- Helps create antibodies
- Improves digestion
- Aids nervous system operation, adrenal gland function, glandular balance

SYMPTOMS AND EFFECTS OF A VITAMIN B$_5$ DEFICIENCY
- Fatigue
- Muscle cramps
- Stomach pain
- Vomiting

NONINFLAMMATORY FOOD SOURCES
- Almonds
- Black beans
- Chickpeas
- Lentils

INTAKE REQUIREMENTS AND SUPPLEMENT RECOMMENDATIONS
- RDI: 10 mg
- No observed adverse effects level: 1,000 mg
- Acne-Free recommendation: 10 to 250 mg

Vitamin B$_6$ (Pyridoxine)

FEATURES AND BENEFITS

- Required for function of more than sixty enzymes
- Essential for processing amino acids
- Helps in the formation of several neurotransmitters
- Essential for regulation of mental processes that influence mood
- Lowers homocysteine levels—a substance linked to cardiovascular disease, stroke, osteoporosis, and Alzheimer's disease (in combination with folic acid and B$_{12}$)
- Helps synthesize fatty acids
- Helps metabolize cholesterol
- Used to produce neurotransmitters, including serotonin, melatonin, and dopamine
- Crucial for a healthy immune system
- Maintains blood sugar within a normal range

SYMPTOMS AND EFFECTS OF A VITAMIN B$_6$ DEFICIENCY

- Dermatitis
- Glossitis (sore tongue)
- Depression
- Confusion
- Convulsions

NONINFLAMMATORY FOOD SOURCES

- Eggs
- Lentils
- Pinto beans
- Salmon

INTAKE REQUIREMENTS AND SUPPLEMENT RECOMMENDATIONS

- RDI: 2 mg
- No observed adverse effects level: 200 mg
- Acne-Free recommendation: 50 to 100 mg

Vitamin B_{12} (Cyanocobalamin)

FEATURES AND BENEFITS

- Functions in the gastrointestinal tract, the nervous system, and the bone marrow
- Helps maintain healthy nerve cells and red blood cells
- Needed to make DNA
- Lowers homocysteine levels (in combination with folic acid and B_6)

SYMPTOMS AND EFFECTS OF A VITAMIN B_{12} DEFICIENCY

- Pernicious anemia
- Fatigue
- Weakness
- Nausea
- Constipation
- Flatulence
- Loss of appetite
- Weight loss
- Numbness and tingling in the hands and feet

NONINFLAMMATORY FOOD SOURCES

- Eggs
- Halibut
- Salmon
- Yogurt

INTAKE REQUIREMENTS AND SUPPLEMENT RECOMMENDATIONS

- RDI: 6 mcg
- No observed adverse effects level: 3,000 mcg
- Acne-Free recommendation: 5 to 100 mcg
- *Special Note:* Deficiency often occurs in strict vegetarians who eat no animal products

Folic Acid (Folate)

FEATURES AND BENEFITS

- Necessary for synthesis of nucleic acids
- Aids in the formation of red blood cells
- Lowers homocysteine levels (in combination with B_{12} and B_6)

SYMPTOMS AND EFFECTS OF A FOLIC ACID DEFICIENCY

- Insufficient and enlarged red blood cells (megaloblastic anemia)
- Gastrointestinal problems
- Sore tongue
- Cracks at corners of mouth
- Diarrhea
- Ulceration of stomach and intestines

NONINFLAMMATORY FOOD SOURCES

- Asparagus
- Avocado
- Beet
- Black beans
- Brussels sprouts
- Cauliflower
- Chickpeas
- Dried beans
- Kale
- Kidney beans
- Melon
- Parsnips
- Spinach

INTAKE REQUIREMENTS AND SUPPLEMENT RECOMMENDATIONS

- RDI: 400 mcg
- No observed adverse effects level: 1,000 mcg
- Acne-Free recommendation: 400 to 800 mcg

Biotin

FEATURES AND BENEFITS

- Helps metabolism of fats, carbohydrates, and proteins
- Aids in utilization of folic acid, vitamin B_5, and vitamin B_1
- Promotes healthy hair

SYMPTOMS AND EFFECTS OF A BIOTIN DEFICIENCY

- Anorexia
- Nausea
- Vomiting
- Inflammation of the tongue
- Gray pallor
- Depression
- Hair loss
- Dermatitis

INTAKE REQUIREMENTS AND SUPPLEMENT RECOMMENDATIONS

- RDI: 300 mcg (Note: Biotin supplements should be taken when the daily intake of alpha lipoic acid exceeds 100 mg. This is because alpha lipoic acid can compete with biotin and in the long run, interfere with biotin's activities in the body.)
- No observed adverse effects level: 2,500 mcg
- Acne-Free recommendation: 300 mcg

Vitamin C

Vitamin C is another superstar in the pantheon of antioxidant acne fighters. There are two basic types of vitamin C, and each makes important contributions.

The form of vitamin C with which people are most familiar is L-ascorbic acid, which is water soluble. As a water-soluble vitamin, L-ascorbic acid protects the cytosol, the watery interior of the cell.

But there is a fat-soluble form of vitamin C called vitamin C ester. (The best known vitamin C ester—and the ester I prescribe for topical use—is ascorbyl palmitate.) Vitamin C ester protects the fatty portions of the cell, which are not protected by L-ascorbic acid.

Vitamin C: One Kind for Your Inside, Another for Your Outside

There is much confusion about a fat-soluble form of vitamin C called vitamin C ester. An ester is simply a chemical compound that combines an acid and an alcohol. Ascorbyl palmitate—the best known ester of vitamin C—is made by adding a fatty acid from palm oil to L-ascorbic acid. The resulting chemical bond creates a fat-soluble compound that contains vitamin C.

Ascorbyl palmitate protects the critical cell membranes in skin tissue. Esters like ascorbyl palmitate should be the vitamin C forms of choice for skin care products because they are absorbed and retained by the skin substantially better than L-ascorbic acid.

Vitamin C (L-Ascorbic Acid and Ascorbyl Palmitate)

Vitamin C is ascorbic acid, a water-soluble compound. Ascorbyl palmitate is ascorbic acid bonded to a fatty acid to make a fat-soluble delivery system for vitamin C.

FEATURES AND BENEFITS
- Water-soluble (L-ascorbic acid) or fat-soluble (vitamin C esters like ascorbyl palmitate)
- Promotes collagen production
- Essential for functioning of neurotransmitters, including dopamine, serotonin, and acetylcholine
- Accumulates inside white blood cells to maintain strong immune response
- Defends against free radicals in the skin created by sunlight, ozone, and harsh chemicals
- Accumulates in the central nervous system to fight free radical activity.

Scurvy: Not Just in Sailors

Vitamin C deficiencies are much more common than many doctors believe. In 1997, a University of Arizona team led by researcher Carol Johnston, Ph.D., tested blood samples from a random group of 494 middle-income people. The tests showed that 30 percent were vitamin C-depleted, and 6.3 percent suffered from the more severe condition called vitamin C deficiency, which produces the symptoms of a disease once called scurvy, that afflicted sailors and others deprived of fresh fruits and vegetables for long periods.

Vitamin C is the foundation of my antioxidant program, but it is also a fragile, unstable nutrient. Since the vitamin C levels in our foods are affected by climate, soil conditions, storage time, temperature, and cooking, it is impossible to tell exactly how much vitamin C you are actually getting at mealtime—hence the wisdom of taking 500 to 1,000 milligrams of supplemental vitamin C a day.

SYMPTOMS AND EFFECTS OF A VITAMIN C DEFICIENCY
- Scurvy
- Parkinson's disease
- Loss of muscle tone
- Loss of sense of well-being
- Wrinkles
- Weakened immunity; increased susceptibility to infections

INTAKE REQUIREMENTS AND SUPPLEMENT RECOMMENDATIONS
- RDI: 60 mg
- No observed adverse effects level: 1,000 mg or more
- Acne-Free recommendation: 1,000 mg ascorbic acid and 500 mg ascorbyl palmitate

The RDI of 60 mg is inadequate to provide the antioxidant action that vitamin C offers or to maintain reasonable levels in skin tissues. Even if you take the higher oral doses I recommend, you will need to use cosmetics that contain a vitamin C ester such as ascorbyl palmitate to attain vitamin C skin levels high enough to reduce inflammation effectively.

To avoid gastric discomfort and maintain adequate blood levels, divide the dosage into three or four portions a day.

For maximum absorption of the ascorbic acid form, look for capsules of vitamin C or add powered vitamin C crystals to water or tea. (Hard vitamin C tablets tend to pass intact through the digestive tract.) Note: There is good evidence that vitamin C is better absorbed when it is combined with bioflavonoids (anti-inflammatory antioxidants found in citrus and other foods). However, vitamin C products with bioflavonoids do not contain enough of them to produce this effect.

The makers of Ester-C (not to be confused with vitamin C Ester, the fat soluble form of vitamin C) also make superior-absorption claims for their mineral-bound vitamin C product, which also contains vitamin C metabolites (breakdown products). While Ester-C has shown superior absorption in rats and in isolated human cells, the only peer-reviewed human clinical trial showed no absorption advantage.[18] Both Ester-C and vitamin C with bioflavonoids are substantially more costly than plain L-ascorbic acid—a fact that would seem to cancel any moderate increase in bodily absorption or cellular uptake these products may offer.

NONINFLAMMATORY FOOD SOURCES
- Broccoli
- Cantaloupe
- Citrus fruits
- Red bell peppers
- Strawberries
- Tomatoes

Vitamin E: Every Cell's Perimeter Defense

FEATURES AND BENEFITS
- Fat soluble
- Lowers cholesterol

- Reduces blood pressure
- Prevents cataracts
- Decreases risk of stroke
- Enhances immune system
- Decreases symptoms of Alzheimer's disease
- Prevents heart attacks
- Protects cell plasma membrane

NONINFLAMMATORY FOOD SOURCES
- Almonds
- Asparagus
- Hazelnuts
- Olives
- Pecans
- Spinach
- Sunflower seeds

INTAKE REQUIREMENTS AND SUPPLEMENT RECOMMENDATIONS
- RDI: 30 IU
- No observed adverse effects level: 1,200 IU
- Acne-Free recommendation 400 to 800 IU

Vitamin E is composed of eight separate components, which are divided into two groups, four tocopherols and four tocotrienols. To get all the available benefits, I recommend a combination vitamin E supplement that offers a mix of tocotrienols and tocopherols—especially gamma tocopherols. Look for soft gel capsules that contain a total of 400 to 800 IU of vitamin E. Because it is fat soluble, take it with meals for greatest absorption.

Mind Your Minerals

Calcium
With so many women (and an increasing number of men) concerned about bone density, calcium and magnesium are very important minerals. Nothing is more aging than the dowager's hump and bent

spine of advanced osteoporosis or the fragility that results from paper-thin bones. Your mother used to tell you to drink your milk for strong bones, but supplements will also do the trick. As we get older bone density decreases, and I strongly recommend calcium supplementation.

A debate continues over the best form of calcium to take. It all comes down to price. Chelated forms (for example, calcium citrate or malate) are absorbed by the body a bit better but are also noticeably costlier than calcium carbonate—the standard, cheapest form. Calcium carbonate is a good choice unless your digestive system is weak. If it is, take a chelated version, or increase your calcium carbonate intake to account for the lowered absorption level.

FEATURES AND BENEFITS
- Essential for healthy teeth, gums, and bones
- Reduces cholesterol deposits
- Relieves muscle spasms
- Lowers blood pressure
- Relieves PMS in some cases
- Assists in absorption of nutrients across cell membranes
- Aids muscle contraction
- Facilitates nerve conduction

SYMPTOMS AND EFFECTS OF A CALCIUM DEFICIENCY
- Osteoporosis
- Bleeding gums
- Rickets

NONINFLAMMATORY FOOD SOURCES
- Collards, kale, and turnip greens
- Cooked broccoli (cooking makes the calcium more available)
- Nuts and seeds
- Sardines or salmon (canned with bones)
- Sea vegetables (dulse, kelp, etc.)
- Tofu
- Wheat germ
- Yogurt

INTAKE REQUIREMENTS AND SUPPLEMENT RECOMMENDATIONS
- RDI: 1,000
- No observed adverse effects level: 1,500 mg
- Acne-Free recommendation: 1,200 mg

The richest food sources of calcium are sea vegetables (highest concentration per ounce), cheese, and tofu. Milk and milk products (except yogurt) are the next richest sources, but I do not recommend them as primary calcium sources for my adult patients, since they tend to promote inflammation and are difficult for many people to digest. Further, to meet the RDA standards, you must consume at least three eight-ounce glasses of milk or more than five ounces of hard cheese a day—a goal that can be difficult for many adults. Yogurt, dark green leafy vegetables, seeds, and nuts are better choices but must also be consumed in large quantities to reach the RDA levels, so supplementation is a logical strategy for securing adequate daily calcium. I never recommend calcium without its nutritional partner, magnesium.

Chromium

FEATURES AND BENEFITS
- Regulates blood sugar levels
- Helps metabolize body fat
- Lowers cholesterol
- Helps regulate insulin
- Promotes weight loss
- Important in the metabolism of carbohydrates and fats
- Helps to regulate the amount of glucose in the blood
- Is needed for insulin to work properly

SYMPTOMS AND EFFECTS OF A CHROMIUM DEFICIENCY
- Impaired glucose tolerance
- Impaired growth

NONINFLAMMATORY FOOD SOURCES
- Brewer's yeast
- Calves liver

Quick Tip: Take chromium the same time as vitamin C to maximize absorption.

INTAKE REQUIREMENTS AND SUPPLEMENT RECOMMENDATIONS
- RDI: 120 mcg
- No observed adverse effects level: 1,000 mg
- Acne-Free recommendation: 200 mcg chromium polynicotinate

It is estimated that up to one-third of Americans do not consume these minimal levels, given the unpopularity of the two best food sources. I recommend taking 200 mcg of chromium polynicotinate daily as a supplement. (I do not recommend taking chromium in the form of chromium picolinate, which is associated with some safety concerns.)

Magnesium
FEATURES AND BENEFITS
- Regulates blood pressure
- Promotes muscle tone
- Aids healthy bone and tooth development
- Needed for energy production and protein synthesis

SYMPTOMS AND EFFECTS OF A MAGNESIUM DEFICIENCY
- Muscle spasms
- Tremor
- Convulsions
- Mental derangement

NONINFLAMMATORY FOOD SOURCES
- Almonds
- Avocados
- Dried soybeans
- Oatmeal (not instant)
- Peanuts
- Tofu

INTAKE REQUIREMENTS AND SUPPLEMENT RECOMMENDATIONS
- RDI: 400 mg
- No observed adverse effects level: 700 mg
- Acne-Free recommendation: half to equal amounts of magnesium to calcium: 600 to 1,200 mg depending on calcium intake

Keep in mind that cooking can dissolve as much as three quarters of the available mineral, causing it to leach into the pan.

Selenium
FEATURES AND BENEFITS
- Essential in formation of glutathione
- Neutralizes poisons like mercury and arsenic
- Cuts the rate of certain cancers
- Provides anti-inflammatory relief from psoriasis and rheumatoid arthritis
- Protects cells against the effects of free radicals
- Prevents oxidation of unsaturated fatty acids
- Helps with proper heart function
- Needed for proper immune function

NONINFLAMMATORY FOOD SOURCES
- Brazil nuts
- Garlic
- Liver, such as calves liver
- Poultry
- Seafood, both fish and shellfish

INTAKE REQUIREMENTS AND SUPPLEMENT RECOMMENDATIONS
- RDI: 70 mcg
- No observed adverse effects level: 200 mcg
- Acne-Free recommendation: 200 mcg chromium polynicotinate

Zinc
FEATURES AND BENEFITS
- Help wounds heal
- Boosts energy metabolism

- Helps body maintain healthy collagen
- An element of superoxidismutase (SOD), a key free radical fighter
- Essential for normal cell division

SYMPTOMS AND EFFECTS OF A ZINC DEFICIENCY
- Worsening of acne, psoriasis, and eczema

NONINFLAMMATORY FOOD SOURCES
- Brazil nuts
- Chicken
- Halibut
- Oatmeal (not instant)
- Salmon
- Sunflower seeds
- Turkey

INTAKE REQUIREMENTS AND SUPPLEMENT RECOMMENDATIONS
- RDI: 15 mcg
- No observed adverse effects level: 200 mg
- Acne-Free recommendation: 15 to 30 mg

Amino Acids and Nutritional Isolates

The final group of recommended supplements is a mix of antioxidants and nutritional compounds. For some, there are no existing RDAs. I have derived supplement recommendations from published research sources.

L-Carnitine
FEATURES AND BENEFITS
- Allows fats to be transported into the mitochondria for energy
- Promotes weight loss by improving fat metabolism
- Prevents free radical damage

SYMPTOMS AND EFFECTS OF AN L-CARNITINE DEFICIENCY
- Inability to harvest the energy stored in fatty acids and a buildup of fatty intermediates that can prove toxic to cells

- Dairy products
- Meat

- RDI: None established
- No observed adverse effects level: None established
- Acne-Free recommendation: 500 to 1,500 mg, depending on age and health. If you are under thirty years old and feel energetic, you will do well on 500 milligrams. If you have chronic health problems, such as diabetes, heart disease, or chronic fatigue, I advise you to take between 1,000 to 1,500 milligrams. For maximum absorption, divide the doses into three separate portions.

Acetyl L-Carnitine

Another form of carnitine, called acetyl L-carnitine, is available as a supplement. It cannot be derived from food. When scientists add the acetyl portion to the carnitine, it allows the carnitine to pass the blood-brain barrier more readily. Acetyl L-carnitine is therapeutic to brain cells. I have found in my clinical practice that supplementing diets with acetyl L-carnitine tends to accelerate fat loss much better in my patients than L-carnitine alone.

- Improves cognitive function, including memory and problem-solving ability
- Promotes skin health

- RDI: None established
- No observed adverse effects level: None established
- Acne-Free recommendation: 500 to 1,000 mg

Coenzyme Q 10 (CoQ10)
- Fat soluble
- Relieves congestive heart failure

- Reduces angina and high blood pressure
- Increases metabolic efficiency to fight weight gain
- Reduces risk of breast and prostate cancer
- Preserves the antioxidant action of vitamin C
- May prevent atherosclerosis
- Protects both the mitochondria and the cell membrane against oxidative damage
- Strengthens the gums to protect against periodontal disease

SYMPTOMS AND EFFECTS OF A COENZYME Q 10 DEFICIENCY

- CoQ10 deficiency is common in individuals with heart disease. Heart tissue biopsies performed on patients with different types of heart diseases showed a coenzyme Q 10 deficiency in 50 to 75 percent of the cases.
- CoQ10 deficiency can affect brain and nerve function

NONINFLAMMATORY FOOD SOURCES

Only small amounts of coenzyme Q 10 are available in foods. You would have to eat a pound of sardines or two and a half pounds of peanuts to get the minimum daily amount recommended for healthy people. CoQ10 is best taken as a supplement, and optimal absorption occurs when taken with meals. (Note: If you have heart problems, check with your physician for the right dosage of CoQ10 for you.)

INTAKE REQUIREMENTS AND SUPPLEMENT RECOMMENDATIONS

- RDI: None established
- No observed adverse effects level: None established—considered extremely safe for healthy persons even at high doses. While it may be beneficial for diabetes or heart disease, individuals with these conditions should not take CoQ10 except under a doctor's supervision.
- Acne-Free recommendation: 30 to 300 mg

CoQ10 levels tend to drop as you grow older, particularly in postmenopausal women. Since CoQ10 is essential for heart health, some cardiologists believe that the increased incidence of congestive heart failure in women of this age is due in part to the significant drop in their CoQ10 levels.

Glutamine

FEATURES AND BENEFITS

- Heals gastrointestinal tract irritation
- Aids in treating individuals with gastrointestinal diseases, such as Crohn's disease, colitis, short bowel syndrome, and irritable bowel syndrome, who require higher levels of glutamine
- Reduces fatigue
- Increases endurance during exercise
- Helps counteract the effects of alcoholism
- Raises serum glucose levels to fight hypoglycemia
- Aids the liver and the intestines
- Strengthens the immune system
- Preserves muscle tissue
- Stimulates growth hormone release
- Serves as fuel for the heart muscle
- Aids in glutathione production in the cells

NONINFLAMMATORY FOOD SOURCES

- Fish
- Legumes
- Poultry

INTAKE REQUIREMENTS AND SUPPLEMENT RECOMMENDATIONS

- RDI: None established
- No observed adverse effects level: None established
- Acne-Free recommendation: 1,500 mg (500 mg three times a day)

Levels of this protective amino acid fall sharply as you age and during any illness, burn, or trauma. Glutamine is especially helpful for athletes and the aging population. I recommend higher levels for athletes, aging patients, and those who are suffering from acute and chronic diseases. It is extremely effective in healing the GI tract.

OPC (Grape Seed Extract/Pycnogenol)

OPC is the scientific name of an antioxidant complex derived from various plants—especially grape seeds and pine bark. OPC stands for oligomeric proanthocyanidin—a class of extremely potent antioxidant compounds. Many experts believe that the OPCs in red wine explain the French paradox—that is, that the French enjoy relatively low rates of heart disease despite a diet high in saturated fat. OPCs are believed to help prevent the oxidation of blood fats and cholesterol upon which much arterial heart disease is blamed.

OPCs are important to skin care because they protect collagen from free radicals, dampen inflammation, and help maintain the health and integrity of blood vessels. As years go by, capillaries and veins become fragile, resulting in a decline in blood circulation. (In France, grape seed OPC is an approved prescription drug for treating weak blood vessels.) Preserving the blood vessels improves oxygen and food delivery to skin cells, which stimulates their growth and repair.

Consumers can easily become confused by the terminology and competing claims surrounding the two leading supplemental sources of OPCs: grape seed extract and pine bark extract. I recommend taking OPCs in the form of grape seed extract, because the OPC complex found in grape seeds appears to substantially exceed the antioxidant power of the OPC complex found in pine bark. Note: Pine bark extracts are often referred to as "pycnogenol"—the original scientific term for OPCs. However, the term "pycnogenol" is out of common scientific use and is now the registered trademark of a proprietary pine bark extract (Pycnogenol). To avoid confusion, most researchers use the generic term OPC when discussing the antioxidant complexes found in grape seeds and pine bark.

OPCs are also found in berries, grapes, cherries, and wine. OPCs are the main precursors of the blue-violet and red pigments in plants (anthocyanins). Look for reddish-purple capsules to be sure you are getting a concentrated natural product.

FEATURES AND BENEFITS
- Blocks the key enzymes that degrade collagen and other connective tissues
- Neutralizes xanthine oxidase (major generator of free radicals), the potent hydroxyl free radical, and prevents oxidation of body fats and cholesterol
- Now believed to be the key factor in the cardiovascular health-promoting powers of red wine

INTAKE REQUIREMENTS AND SUPPLEMENT RECOMMENDATIONS
- RDI: None established
- No observed adverse effects level: None established
- Acne-Free recommendation: 30 to 100 mg

GLA (Gamma Linolenic Acid)

GLA is an omega-6 essential fatty acid. It is rapidly converted to dihomo-gamma-linolenic acid, the precursor of prostaglandin E1, and a potent anti-inflammatory agent. We become deficient in GLA when large amounts of sugar, trans fatty acids (margarine, hydrogenated oils), red meats, and dairy are consumed.

Very little GLA is found in the average Western diet. Borage oil is the richest supplemental source (17 to 25 percent GLA), followed by black currant oil (15 to 20 percent GLA), and evening primrose oil (EPO) (7 to 10 percent GLA). Borage and evening primrose oils are the most common supplemental sources. GLA should be taken with food, to increase absorption.

FEATURES AND BENEFITS
- Production of prostaglandins
- Prevents hardening of the arteries
- Lowers cholesterol
- Lowers blood pressure
- Inhibits blood clotting
- Reduces blood triglycerides
- Reduces LDL cholesterol levels

- Prevents blockage of arteries
- Enhances die-off of cancer cells
- Suppresses growth of malignant tumors
- Offsets degenerative signs of aging
- May help PMS (weak evidence)
- Reduces benign breast disease, eczema, psoriasis, obesity, and vascular disorders
- Effective to varying degrees in treating arthritis, alcoholism, asthma, diabetic neuropathy, and multiple sclerosis

INTAKE REQUIREMENTS AND SUPPLEMENT RECOMMENDATIONS
- RDI: None established
- No observed adverse effects level: None established
- Acne-Free recommendation: 250 to 1,000 mg

Turmeric

This brilliant yellow spice has been a culinary mainstay in many cultures for thousands of years. Turmeric, a member of the ginger family, is the ingredient that gives Asian curries their characteristic bright-yellow hue. The spice's active compounds are potent anti-inflammatory antioxidant substances called curcuminoids.

FEATURES AND BENEFITS
- Potent antioxidant that prevents free radical formation and neutralizes existing free radicals
- May reduce risk of Alzheimer's disease
- Antiviral, noninflammatory, anticancer effects
- Lowers bad cholesterol
- Treats AIDS by blocking activation of the LTR gene in the HIV's DNA
- Used in India's ancient ayurvedic medicine as a stomach tonic, for cuts, wounds, poor vision, rheumatic pains, coughs, liver disease, and to increase milk production
- Protects the liver

INTAKE REQUIREMENTS AND SUPPLEMENT RECOMMENDATIONS
- RDI: None established
- No observed adverse effects level: None established
- Acne-Free recommendation: 250 to 1,000 mg

Turmeric should be stored in the freezer or refrigerator to keep the volatile oils fresh and active.

The right supplements—the second tier of my acne-free program—are essential in the treatment and prevention of acne. But diet and supplements are not all that are necessary to achieve clear skin. Next, we'll explore the facet of my program that many of my patients say they love the most—topical anti-inflammatories that can clear the skin while increasing radiance and tone.

6

The Three-Tiered Perricone Anti-Acne Program— Tier 3: Topical Anti-Inflammatories

As a dermatologist I am the first to admit to having a long love affair with efficacious topical therapies. When I can give my patients a lotion or cream and know that after only a few applications they will see a radical resolution of their skin problems, I know that all my years of research were well worth it.

Throughout this book I have stressed the role of inflammation in acne—acne is an inflammatory disease. Traditional dermatologists have missed the point in their quest for effective acne treatments. I have explained in previous chapters and will quickly recap here that the so-called primary event, the formation of the comedone or microcomedone, is the result of inflammation. There is solid proof that interleukin-1 can cause the keratinocytes inside the follicle to become sticky, resulting in the following:

- A plug is formed which can lead to an open and/or closed comedone
- Which leads to a cascade of inflammatory chemicals
- Which can cause the comedone to become a papule, pustule, or cyst

Thus, it's not the plugging of the follicle that leads to inflammation, it's inflammation that leads to the plugging of the follicle. Armed with this knowledge, we can now move on to a discussion of powerful therapeutic tools: nutrient-based natural anti-inflammatories that can be applied directly to the skin.

Alpha Lipoic Acid

In the previous chapter, we discussed the importance of the antioxidant alpha lipoic acid and its powerful anti-inflammatory effect. When taken systemically, alpha lipoic acid performs a variety of important functions, such as helping to regulate blood sugar by increasing sensitivity to insulin, at the same time enabling the cells to better utilize sugar and carry it into the cell rather than circulating in the bloodstream.[1-4]

But what happens when we apply alpha lipoic acid topically?

The fat-soluble portion of alpha lipoic acid is of tremendous benefit to the skin. This is because the skin tends to repel anything that contains water or is water soluble. Just put a few drops of water on the back of your hand and watch what happens. Instead of being absorbed into the skin, it runs right off. Substances that are water soluble do not penetrate the skin very well, and that's why I have stressed the importance of fat-soluble molecules for skin treatment, such as vitamin C ester and vitamin E. Alpha lipoic acid is extremely fat soluble. In fact, scientists have found measurable amounts of alpha lipoic acid in both the deeper portions of the skin and the subcutaneous fat within four hours of its topical application in a cream base.[5] Alpha lipoic acid is also intimately involved in the cell's energy production, that is, the conversion of food to energy. When alpha lipoic acid is abundant in the cellular environment, the cell is better able to produce energy and conduct critical functions, including cellular repair.

Such energy production also helps the cell resist the destructive effects of oxidative stress and inflammation. This is particularly important to acne patients, because scientists have observed that the sebaceous glands of acne patients do not function optimally. There are a number of causes for this. One is neuropeptides, as discussed in Chapter 3; another is because decreased levels of energy cause the sebaceous glands to produce abnormal levels of chemicals called triglycerides. When these triglycerides are produced in abnormal ratios within the sebaceous gland, they tend to be proinflammatory, increasing the stickiness of the exfoliating cells, and thus heightening the likelihood of a clogged pore.

DMAE

I have discussed DMAE (dimethylaminoethanol) in my previous books and earlier in this book. The therapeutic effects of the DMAE as it relates to acne and acne scars are impressive. DMAE is a nutritional substance found in fish, especially wild Alaskan salmon. Chemists do not consider DMAE an antioxidant; however it does have powerful anti-inflammatory activities within the cell. The anti-inflammatory activity comes about because DMAE intersperses itself in the outer fatty portion of the cell (the cell plasma membrane). Visualize the walls of your house. Once DMAE is interspersed in the lipid bilayers it acts very much like the reinforcements in the walls of your house. The DMAE prevents the breakdown of the wall, which in turn produces proinflammatory chemicals and precursors—such as arachidonic acid and oxidized fatty acids—much like reinforced walls are better able to withstand the elements of nature that can cause premature breakdown of the house's walls. DMAE can also act as a penetration enhancer, and enhances the anti-inflammatory effects of alpha lipoic acid.

As mentioned in the previous chapters, DMAE is a building block of the neurotransmitter acetylcholine, and may be taken orally as a cognitive enhancer. This wonderful ability to assist levels of the neurotransmitter acetylcholine gives DMAE an important role in the treatment of aging face and body.

Here is how it works. When DMAE is applied to the skin in a penetrating base, within a matter of minutes increased tone is observed. As we know, an aging face and body are characterized not only by wrinkling, but also by sagging. Until the discovery of DMAE, the sags that came with aging could only be corrected by cosmetic surgery. The topical application of DMAE has a cumulative effect. The increased tone that results can actually change the shape of the face and the body over a period of months.

But that's not all. Many of my acne patients are plagued by pimples and unsightly large pores. These large pores can actually absorb foundation makeup, making the skin appear pitted. The same ability that DMAE has to increase tone also actually helps decrease the appearance of large pores over a period of a couple of weeks. When DMAE is applied daily, even patients with the largest pores develop a porcelain-like appearance to their skin within a matter of weeks.

DMAE's powerful anti-inflammatory activity, in addition to its superior abilities as a penetration enhancer, results in the reduction of visible acne inflammation within twenty-four to forty-eight hours. When used in combination with alpha lipoic acid, DMAE enhances the scar prevention and treatment aspects of alpha lipoic acid. In my own office, I conducted a study using topical alpha lipoic acid and DMAE with fifteen patients suffering from atrophic (indented) acne scars. The patients were directed to apply the combination alpha lipoic acid/DMAE cream to their facial scars twice daily. Patients were photographed at the beginning of the study and then re-photographed on a monthly basis. At the end of a six-month period, the fifteen patients showed an 80 percent reduction in the severity of their acne scars. The efficacy of this topical combination is quite surprising considering that acne scars are traditionally treated with lasers, dermabrasion, and other more extreme surgical procedures that yield far less visible benefits than this combination of two potent topicals.

Another even more impressive study was conducted on the alpha lipoic acid/DMAE combination for the treatment of postsurgical scars. A double-blind placebo study was conducted by plastic surgeons on children following cleft lip and palate surgical repair.[6] Children who undergo this surgery usually end up with scars above their upper lips, which causes some deformity of the mouths. Parents were given either a lotion containing alpha lipoic acid and DMAE in a penetrating base, or the penetrating base alone, which contained no active ingredients. In this study, the parents were instructed to apply the lotion twice daily to the surgical site. The children's surgeons examined their patients postoperatively at three-month intervals. The important aspect of a controlled double-blind placebo study is that neither the doctor nor the subject (in this case, the parent) knows whether they are using the active agent or the placebo. This ensures an objective observation of the efficacy of the treatment. At the end of one year, final photographs were taken of the patients, and the code on the treatment bottles was deciphered. The children who had received the twice-daily application of alpha lipoic acid and DMAE combination had almost no visible scar—and no upper lip deformity. The children who had received the placebo had obvious scarring and deformity and showed no benefit whatsoever.

The results of this study are important because they illustrate that we can prevent serious scarring and accompanying deformity. And, because the findings were achieved through a double-blind controlled study, the conclusions carry more weight with scientists than do open studies (as in the case of the atrophic acne scar study noted earlier).

DMAE is a miracle nutrient in that it can act as a cognitive enhancer; an anti-aging topical; and a therapeutic tool for the treatment of acne, acne scars, and other types of scars. DMAE offers many benefits, both cosmetic and therapeutic, to anyone interested in beauty and health.

Glutathione

Glutathione is a powerful antioxidant found in all our body's cells. It is a water-soluble antioxidant that is made up of three amino acids: cysteine, glycine, and glutamic acid; therefore, it is called a tripeptide. Glutathione contains a sulfur molecule attached to hydrogen (a molecular combination called the thiol group) and is an important component in cellular respiration. The most important antioxidant that our cells produce is glutathione. I will recap some of the basic science here so that you can get a really clear idea of the importance of glutathione and how it fits into the overall picture.

As my readers know, the body's antioxidant defense systems are critical to maintaining health and preserving beauty. Antioxidants are our defense against destructive molecules called free radicals. Simply stated, the majority of free radicals are derived from oxygen, hence the term "antioxidant." Free radicals are generated by normal metabolism, that is, conversion of food to energy. They are also generated in the cell by external sources such as toxins, ultraviolet radiation, and other stressors. When free radicals attack the outer portion of the cell, (the cell plasma membrane), they tend to oxidize fats and activate enzymes, resulting in the flow of proinflammatory chemicals into the cell. Thus, the free radicals create inflammation. To compound the problem, the inflammation then goes on to trigger the production of even more free radicals (a cascade). Once an inflammatory cascade has begun, glutathione is quickly depleted, leading to even greater inflammation. In order to prevent the destructive effects of inflammation from free radicals, powerful antioxidants such as glutathione enable other antioxidants—anti-inflammatories such as vitamin C and vitamin E—to protect all portions of the cell, both the fat-soluble cell plasma membrane and the water-soluble portion of the cell known as the cytosol.

In the fight against inflammation caused by free radicals, scientists look at the balance between antioxidants and free radicals. As we have mentioned before, this balance is known as the "redox" status of the cell. The redox status is the ratio of oxidants (bad guys) to reducing agents (good guys) within the cells. If cells do not maintain the correct redox balance, proinflammatory chemicals are created. When these are released they cause severe damage on all levels, leading to virtually every disease process we can think of, from acne and Alzheimer's disease to diabetes and cancer. Glutathione plays a critical, essential role in maintaining redox balance in the cell, as it interacts with other antioxidants, such as vitamin E, vitamin C, as well as coenzyme Q 10, assisting their function in protecting the cell.[7] It is critical to maintain adequate levels of glutathione within the cell to prevent the accumulation of inflammatory chemicals, which trigger the activation of transcription factors such as NfkB. This is important for acne patients because these transcription factors trigger production of cytokines such as interleukin-1, which causes abnormal exfoliation within the follicle by making the cells known as keratinocytes sticky. The result is retention hyperkeratosis, which results in a clogged pore. And the next step after a pore is clogged is the formation of the microcomedone and comedones—the birth of an acne lesion.

Glutathione is also an important detoxifying agent, enabling the body to eliminate toxins and poisons. Glutathione regulates and regenerates our immune cells and thus modulates the inflammatory response in the vicinity of the acne lesion.

Glutathione also protects enzyme proteins that inhibit collagen-digesting enzymes that cause damage to the skin in or around acne lesions. As you recall, it is the collagen-digesting enzymes that break down the collagen within the dermis, resulting in acne scars. It must be emphasized again that it is critical to have adequate amounts of glutathione in all of our cells to regulate the redox status and inflammation at the site of the acne lesions.[8]

Glutathione can be applied once daily to clinically normal skin or to active skin lesions. Due to the sulfur content of its thiol group, glutathione possesses some antibacterial activity. The sulfur content can also cause some peeling of the acne lesions, which helps clear plugged follicles. When glutathione is applied to acne lesions—open or closed comedones, or clinically inflamed lesions such as papules, pustules, and cysts—the results are rapidly observed. In fact, application of glutathione causes an immediate reduction in obvious lesions, and thus can be used as a spot treatment. We're all familiar with stress pimples that seem to show up (usually in some impossible-to-miss spot!) just when we're getting ready for a special occasion. I have created a special glutathione formula for my patients in a tinted base cream that has a twofold function. First, the tint conceals the redness of the inflammatory lesions. Second, the glutathione rapidly reduces the inflammation, imparting both cosmetic and therapeutic benefits.

After experiencing the efficacy of topical glutathione on their acne lesions, my patients often ask whether glutathione would be just as effective if taken orally. Unfortunately, the answer is no. Because glutathione is a tripeptide (composed of three amino acids), it is rapidly digested in the gastrointestinal system, and its therapeutic activity is destroyed. I do, however, advise my patients that the precursors, or building blocks, of glutathione may be taken orally in capsules containing N-acetyl cysteine and alpha lipoic acid that work synergistically to elevate the cells' glutathione levels, providing maximum antioxidant and anti-inflammatory reserves.

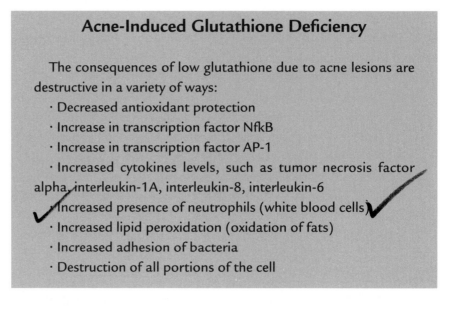

Acne-Induced Glutathione Deficiency

The consequences of low glutathione due to acne lesions are destructive in a variety of ways:
- Decreased antioxidant protection
- Increase in transcription factor NfkB
- Increase in transcription factor AP-1
- Increased cytokines levels, such as tumor necrosis factor alpha, interleukin-1A, interleukin-8, interleukin-6
- Increased presence of neutrophils (white blood cells)
- Increased lipid peroxidation (oxidation of fats)
- Increased adhesion of bacteria
- Destruction of all portions of the cell

Ben's Story

Ben first came to see me when he was a seventeen-year-old high school senior. He had been suffering from acne since the age of fourteen, and three years later it showed no signs of clearing up anytime soon. Ben had been to two other dermatologists, who had treated him with oral and topical antibiotics, as well as various topical treatments including retinoids and benzoyl peroxide. But his acne persisted.

As I was taking Ben's medical history I noted that he appeared to be in excellent physical condition. Ben told me that although he had played on his high school football team, his favorite sports were weight lifting and bodybuilding. Ben's large shoulders, thick neck, and muscular arms were evidence of his devotion to these sports. Further discussion revealed that these recreational sports had become a way of life for Ben; he followed a strict health and fitness regimen both in and out of the gym. Like many bodybuilders, Ben ate a diet extremely high in protein—he consumed approximately 150 to 200 grams of protein per day. The types of protein he favored were primarily from animal sources, consisting of red meat and poultry. He also drank protein powder shakes containing milk proteins, whey, and some soy. Although Ben ate some vegetables, the amount was minuscule, and his overall intake of carbohydrates was extremely low. He also religiously trimmed all the fat and skin from his red meat and poultry and scrupulously avoided fats and oils, in order to follow an extremely low-fat diet. He believed this type of eating was necessary for his bodybuilding program, which consisted of lifting weights six days a week for approximately two hours per day.

In addition to his schoolwork and weight lifting, Ben held a part-time job at the local grocery store, unloading trucks and stacking the warehouse shelves with heavy cases of food. "I like to think of it as pumping groceries," he said with a grin.

Ben's physical examination revealed papules, pustules, and comedoes on his forehead, cheeks, and chin. His upper chest, shoulders, and back were also marked with pustules and papules. His previous dermatologist had started Ben on oral minocycline combined with topical benzoyl peroxide wash and topical clindamycin—all of which he was still using. I observed that there was some well-demarcated redness and dryness apparent on his face, back, and shoulders, caused by the proinflammatory effects of the topical medication. Ben had bright blue eyes, blond hair, and the accompanying light complexion, which made him all the more susceptible to the drying effects of these medications (olive skin with a more oily complexion is better able to tolerate the harsh proinflammatory effects of these types of topicals).

I explained to Ben that the very sport that helped to keep him healthy and fit was contributing to his acne. It is the rule rather than the exception for bodybuilders and weight lifters (as well other types of serious athletes) to suffer from acne flare-ups. Weight lifting, for example, causes an increase in testosterone production, which may exacerbate acne. Ben did not realize that a high-protein, low-carbohydrate, no-fat/low-fat diet is extremely proinflammatory and can also result in both the onset and worsening of acne. He did make an interesting connection, however: he stated that although he had reached puberty at the age of twelve, his acne had not begun until he started lifting weights at age fourteen and a half. At that time, the older guys at the gym recommended that Ben follow a restricted diet to maintain low body fat. He followed their advice and went on to become a competitive bodybuilder. He had won several trophies over the past three years.

Although many athletes, especially those in the fiercely competitive world of bodybuilding, believe they have to follow an extreme diet as outlined above, I explained to Ben that he could maintain the low body fat and significant muscle mass he desired without having to cut out all fats and carbohydrates. I was not surprised at Ben's skeptical reaction. However, he was desperate to do something—anything that could get rid of the severe acne lesions that constantly plagued him. He was all the more motivated by a certain young woman whom he had seen around school. He just didn't have the nerve to approach her with his face covered in angry red pimples.

I immediately placed Ben on the 28-Day Anti-Acne Diet. I enlarged the serving sizes to meet the demands of his extreme workout regimen. I also instructed him to drink at least eight to ten glasses of water a day. I started him on nutritional supplements containing the complete B-complex, calcium, magnesium, DMAE, alpha lipoic acid, N-acetyl cysteine, coenzyme Q 10, and vitamin E in the form of both gamma tocopherols and tocotrienols. The supplements also contained zinc, selenium, and the proper ratio of essential fatty acids such as omega-3s and GLA (gamma linoleic acid).

It was now time to tackle the carbohydrate–no fat issue. Convincing bodybuilders to change their strange diets is one of the greatest challenges in my practice. And yet if Ben was serious about getting rid of his acne he needed to make serious dietary changes. He couldn't have it both ways. I emphasized the importance of eating a well-balanced diet including lots of fruits and vegetables. These foods are rich in antioxidants, which act as natural anti-inflammatories. Fortunately, Ben did not have a problem eliminating sugars and starches from his diet, as he already scrupulously avoided them on his low-carb, high-protein, low-fat diet. Half the battle was won. Now came the hardest part. I told Ben that he needed to incorporate essential fatty acids into his daily meal plan. This included eating fish such as wild Alaskan salmon and taking essential fatty acid supplements two to three times per day.

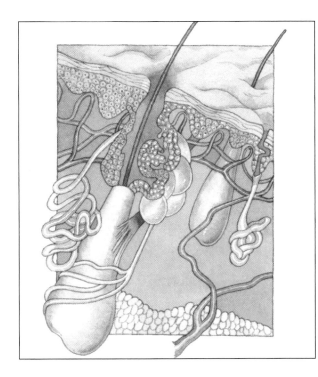

Normal anatomy

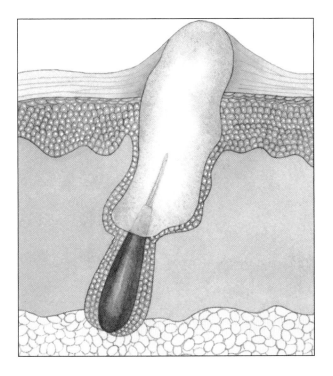

Inflammatory lesion: pustule

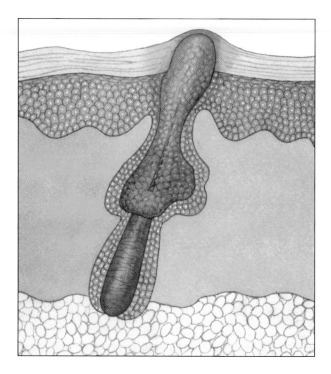

INFLAMMATORY LESION:
papule (pimple)

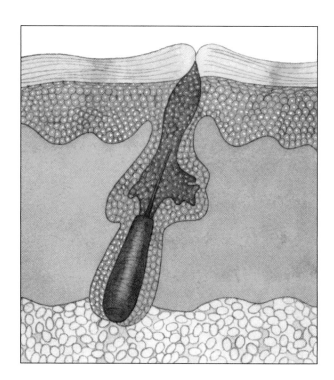

NO MICROSCOPIC
INFLAMMATION VISIBLE:
whitehead (closed comedo)

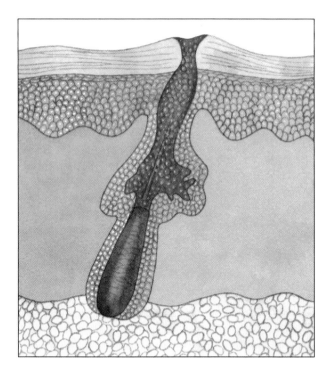

No microscopic
inflammation visible:
blackhead (open comedo)

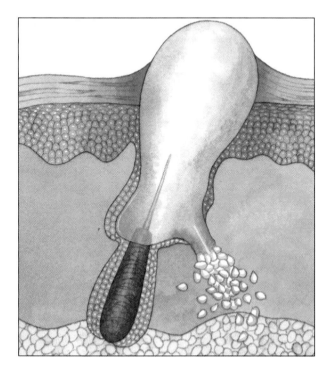

Inflammatory lesion:
nodule (cyst)

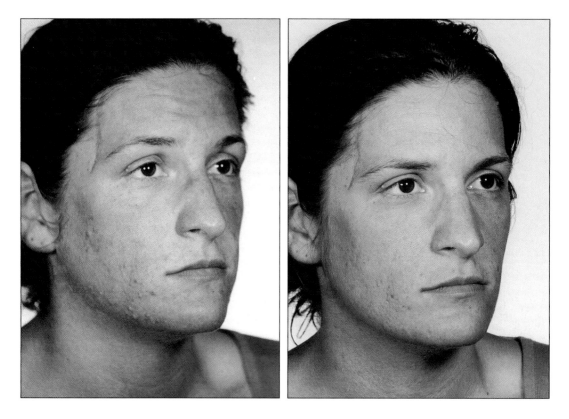

BEFORE: Notice the papules on the jaw line extending up to the cheek, and the redness on the bridge of the nose and cheek area. (Photo: King Vincent Storm Photography)

AFTER: After five days on the program, note the resolution of pustules and papules. Also note the dramatic decrease of redness on the nose. (Photo: King Vincent Storm Photography)

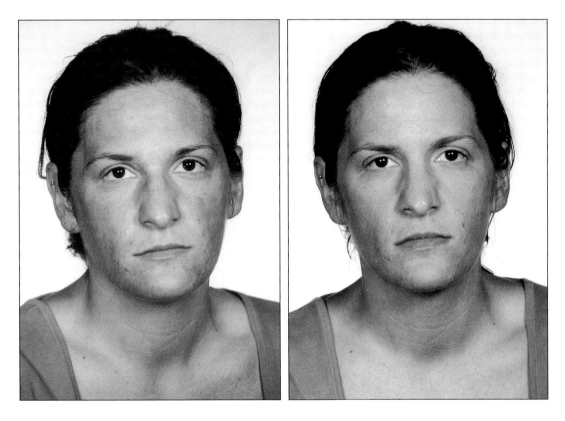

BEFORE: Note the pronounced redness on the bridge of the nose, cheek, and jaw line. Also note the lesions on both cheeks. (Photo: King Vincent Storm Photography)

AFTER: After five days on the program there is a marked decrease in redness and lesions are resolved. (Photo: King Vincent Storm Photography)

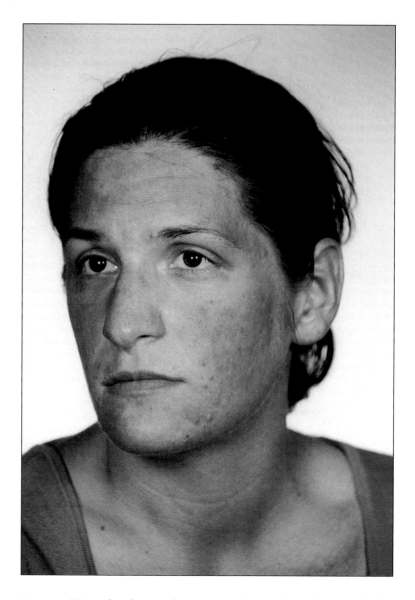

BEFORE: Note the deep redness, pustules, and papules on cheek and jaw area. (Photo: King Vincent Storm Photography)

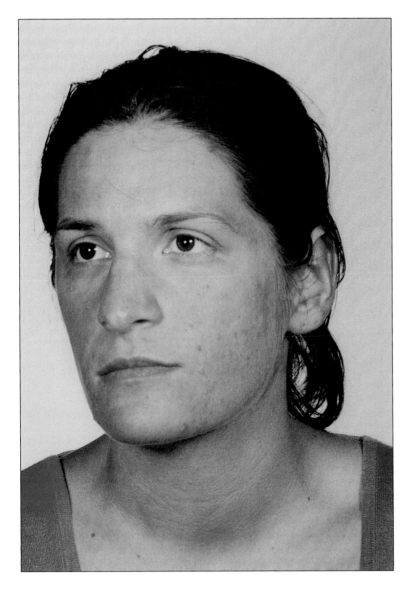

AFTER: After five days on the program, the redness is resolved as well as the majority of lesions. (Photo: King Vincent Storm Photography)

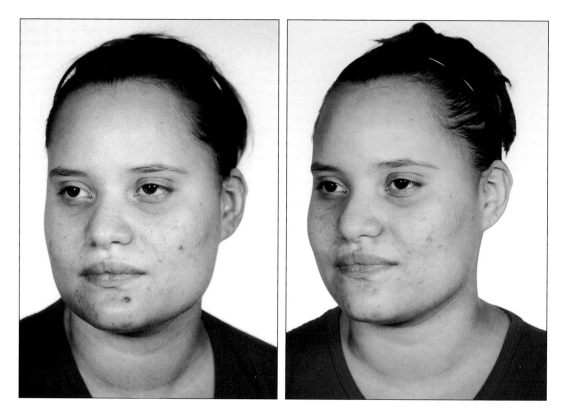

Before: This face is characterized by mild cystic acne with lesions on the chin and cheek area. (Photo: King Vincent Storm Photography)

After: After five days on the program, note the resolution of the large lesions on the chin and cheek. (Photo: King Vincent Storm Photography)

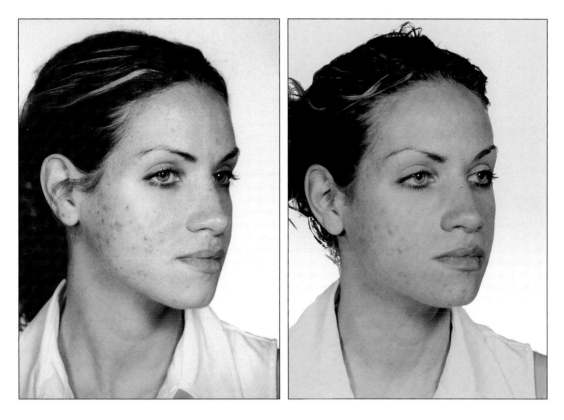

BEFORE: This patient has multiple red papules on the right cheek area and above her upper lip. (Photo: King Vincent Storm Photography)

AFTER: After five days on the program, note the marked decrease in both the redness on the cheek and the number of papules on the cheek and upper lip. (Photo: King Vincent Storm Photography)

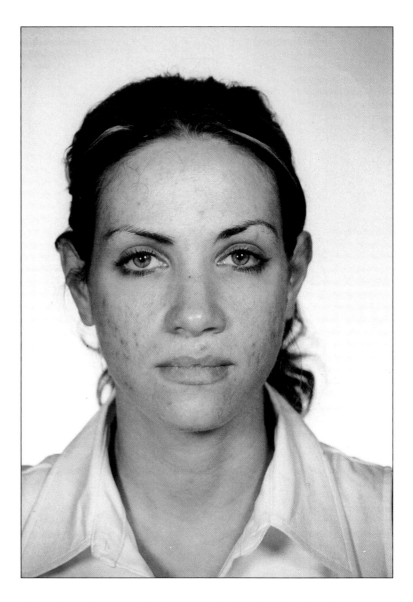

Note the redness and lesions on cheeks, forehead, and upper lip. (Photo: King Vincent Storm Photography)

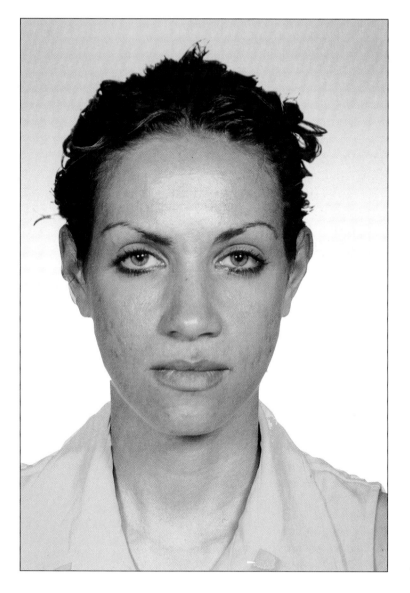

AFTER: Note the complete resolution of redness (erythema) in this subject's skin, following 28 days on the three-tiered anti-inflammatory program.

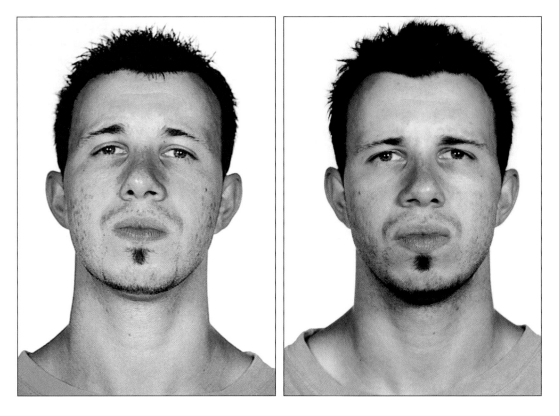

BEFORE: Note the redness across the bridge of the nose and spreading out into the cheek area. (Photo: King Vincent Storm Photography)

AFTER: This photo is important because it illustrates the powerful anti-inflammatory effect of the three-tiered program. Note the dramatic, marked reduction of redness across the bridge of the nose. (Photo: King Vincent Storm Photography)

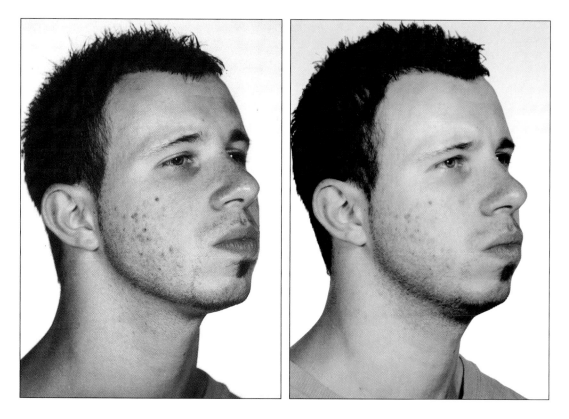

BEFORE: This patient has marked visible inflammatory lesions on the right cheek extending down to his beard area. (Photo: King Vincent Storm Photography)

AFTER: Note the resolution of redness, bumps, and lesions after five days on the program. (Photo: King Vincent Storm Photography)

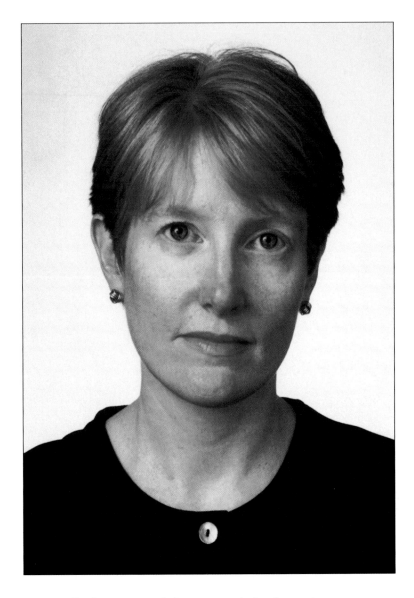

BEFORE: Redness around the nose and cheek area is characteristic of a generalized inflammation that is seen with inflammatory problems like rosacea, seborrahic dermatitis, and acne.

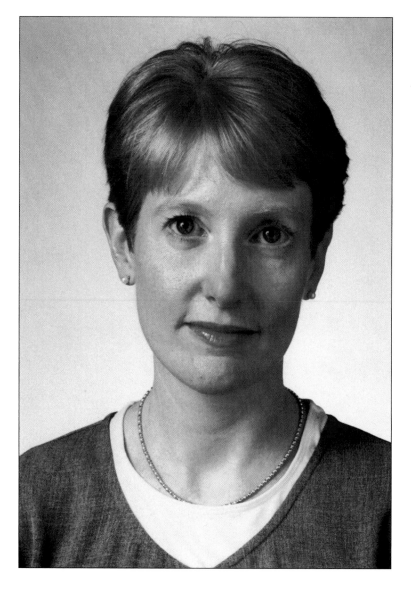

AFTER: After five days on the program, note the marked resolution of papules and redness on the patient's cheeks, chin, upper lip, and forehead. (Photo: King Vincent Storm Photography)

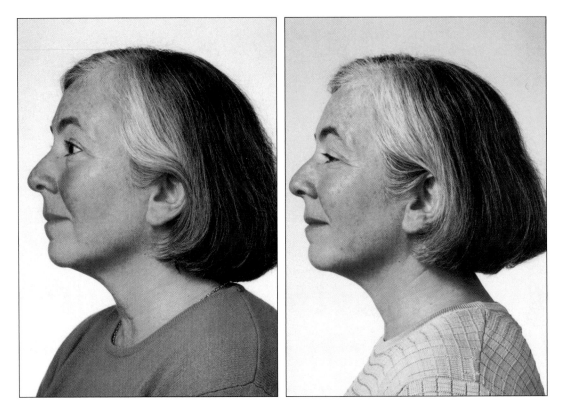

BEFORE: Note the diffused redness (erythema) in the cheek and nose area.

AFTER: After following 28-day three-tiered anti-inflammatory program, profound changes may be noted in this subject's skin: the complete resolution of the underlying redness, and the fading of the erythema in the nose and cheek area.

Ben's Topical Regimen

I gave Ben a cleanser containing DMAE, which acts as both a natural anti-inflammatory and a penetration enhancer. After using the cleanser, Ben was to use toner pads that were saturated with DMAE, alpha lipoic acid, and alpha hydroxy acid. The next step was to apply a gel containing benzoyl peroxide (a traditional acne treatment) in conjunction with topical alpha lipoic acid. Last, I gave Ben a high-potency spot-treatment product containing glutathione, alpha lipoic acid, and DMAE to apply directly to individual lesions and papules as necessary. Ben was concerned when I recommended that he discontinue his current regimen of antibiotics, but he agreed to follow my recommendations for a trial period and return in a month.

I knew that adjusting Ben's diet by incorporating essential fatty acids in the proper ratio, maintaining adequate protein levels, and ensuring adequate levels of antioxidant rich fruits and vegetables with high levels of antioxidants, would soon show visible results. In addition, Ben would be taking a nutritional supplement containing high levels of natural antioxidant, anti-inflammatories, as well as two daily capsules of N-acetyl cysteine and alpha lipoic acids capsules, to provide adequate precursors of glutathione in his cells. This, too, would make a big difference in the clinical course of Ben's acne. It is necessary to pursue an aggressive three-tiered approach of diet, supplements, and topicals with someone like Ben, because anyone who exercises strenuously tends to produce higher levels of androgens, which tend to exacerbate acne.

Finally, drinking eight to ten glasses of water a day is an absolute must. When one is partially dehydrated, there is an increase in the inflammatory chemicals in the cell, resulting in a proinflammatory state. Dehydration also has a dramatic effect on the natural desquamation process of the stratum corneum, a process that is already dysfunctional in acne sufferers. Time and again in my practice I have seen how a simple increase in water intake can decrease onset and severity of acne lesion flare-ups.

I was looking forward to seeing Ben for his follow-up visit four weeks later, as I was convinced that I would see some visible improvement. However, when the day came, I learned that Ben had canceled his appointment. I tried calling Ben but was only able to reach his answering machine. When he returned my call several days later, Ben told me that he'd canceled his appointment because of (as I'd suspected) his busy schedule. However, the good news is that Ben felt no compunction for missing our appointment because he looked and felt terrific. In fact, he didn't feel that a follow-up visit was even necessary! Ben told me that his energy levels had increased, making his weight lifting routines seem easier than before. He'd even increased the weights on a number of his exercises. Best of all, Ben discovered the age-old yet almost impossible-to-believe truth—despite the fact that he had incorporated much more fat into his diet, he was actually leaner than when I had first seen him a little over a month ago!

And now, the final question: what about the acne? Ben's existing lesions had significantly decreased in size and redness. New lesions were not forming the way they used to and the older lesions were resolving at a much quicker rate. Yes, Ben still had acne, but large areas on his face and back were clear for the first time in more than four years. Ben was definitely on the road to a permanent recovery. I asked Ben to follow up with me in approximately three to four weeks for a clinical examination and reevaluation of treatment (and, I told him, no excuses this time). I knew that as Ben's inflammation levels stayed low, and his glutathione and other critical nutrients, such as the essential fatty-acids, increased on a cellular level, his immune system would block the course of this disease.

Putting It All Together

You don't need a shopping bag full of products to treat acne. But, because it is a systemic, inflammatory disease, we must take a systemic, whole-body approach to its treatment. This means starting with and sticking to the anti-inflammatory diet, adding N-acetyl cysteine, alpha lipoic acid, zinc, and essential fatty acids to a well-balanced nutritional supplement regimen and using targeted topical treatments. After cleansing I recommend toning the skin with pads saturated with a toner that contains high levels of DMAE. Follow with products containing the unbeatable combination of alpha lipoic acid and DMAE to clear the skin, provide toning and firming benefits, increase radiance, and fight and prevent scarring. Finally, remember glutathione. Use it as a spot treatment on existing acne lesions and keep your cells well fortified by taking N-acetyl cysteine along with alpha lipoic acid.

There are many different causes of and contributors to acne, but remember what was said in the chapter on stress and acne: regardless of the precipitator, all pathways lead to inflammation. If we can control the inflammation we can control the acne. It really is that simple.

7

Acne and Exercise—
The Long-Term Solution for
Keeping Your Body *and* Your
Face Toned and Clear

As you've learned in the preceding chapters, if you suffer from acne—whether an occasional breakout or chronic, progressive lesions—eliminating it is a multilayered task. One must treat the entire body. Everyone knows that moderate exercise is a vital component of a healthy lifestyle, and this is especially true for the acne patient. We do well to listen to good old-fashioned common sense: moderation is key.

Why? Remember my patient Lisa? As her case illustrated, exercising for too long or too strenuously can worsen your breakouts.

The Perricone Program recommends blending three distinct types of exercise:

- Weight resistance
- Cardiovascular/aerobic
- Flexibility

But acne is unique—much of what might be considered beauty- and health-promoting activities for people without acne can spell disaster for those with acne. Even worse, certain forms of exercise can actually cause or exacerbate acne. Let's take a look at these statements and evaluate them.

Like me, many of my patients, both male and female, practice weight training and/or weight lifting. I first began weight lifting when I was in my teens, and I loved the positive effects it had on my strength and appearance. This motivated me to add a good cardiovascular workout to my exercise routine, and so I began running.

The physical results were great. I became stronger and healthier; my endurance and stamina increased with each passing day. But all was not good news. My newfound fitness and robust, healthy appearance were restricted to my body only. My complexion was another story. I was loath to admit it, but the weight lifting actually made my acne worse. Unfortunately, it is a well-known fact of life among bodybuilders and weight lifters, regardless of gender, that this type of exercise makes the body much more susceptible to acne breakouts. The reason is simple: weight lifting and weight training increases levels of male hormones, such as testosterone. As we learned in Chapter 3, male hormones can contribute to acne.

I should mention flexibility here, too. Cardiovascular aerobic exercises and weight training or weight lifting offer many important benefits to the body, but none of these types of exercises increase flexibility. This is important because as we age our flexibility decreases dramatically. If you doubt this, just spend a few moments watching a child or teenager play, dance, participate in sports, and so on. You'll notice their ease of motion, quickness of response, physical fluidity.

So how can one attain a fit, toned, and flexible body as well as clear, radiant skin at any age? Yoga.

In my opinion, the benefits of yoga are unparalleled. Yoga is unique in that it addresses the entire person.

- It exercises and tones the body.
- It energizes and soothes the mind.
- It helps the practitioner to achieve a deeply meditative state.

Because acne is aggravated by stress, meditation or some form of effective relaxation is necessary to lower stress levels. Yoga provides just that; it is a superior form of meditation. But yoga is not a passive meditation. A twenty-minute yoga session will leave you completely relaxed, physically invigorated, and enjoying a strong sense of well-being. It is the perfect exercise for people who lead busy, stress-filled lives who want to look and feel their best.

To really showcase the many benefits of yoga I went to the experts. Trisha Lamb Feuerstein of the International Association of Yoga Therapists has kindly given me permission to reprint the "Health Benefits of Yoga" that appears on their excellent and informative website at www.iayt.org/benefits.html.

HEALTH BENEFITS OF YOGA

Trisha Lamb Feuerstein

HEALTH BENEFITS

This information is grouped into three categories—physiological benefits, psychological benefits, biochemical effects—and is based on the regular practice of traditional *asana, pranayama,* and meditation. Please note that pulse rate, etc., may increase during the practice of various asanas, some forms of *pranayama,* and some stages of meditation, but overall benefits to general health are as listed below. For information on the physiological changes that occur during the practice of specific asanas, etc., please see James Funderburk's *Science Studies Yoga* and other resources cited at the end of this article.

PHYSIOLOGICAL BENEFITS
- Stable autonomic nervous system equilibrium, with a tendency toward parasympathetic nervous system dominance rather than the usual stress-induced sympathetic nervous system dominance
- Pulse rate decreases
- Respiratory rate decreases
- Blood pressure decreases (of special significance for hyporeactors)

- Galvanic skin response (GSR) increases
- EEG—alpha waves increase (theta, delta, and beta waves also increase during various stages of meditation)
- EMG activity decreases
- Cardiovascular efficiency increases
- Respiratory efficiency increases (respiratory amplitude and smoothness increase, tidal volume increases, vital capacity increases, breath-holding time increases)
- Gastrointestinal function normalizes
- Endocrine function normalizes
- Excretory functions improve
- Musculoskeletal flexibility and joint range of motion increase
- Posture improves
- Strength and resiliency increase
- Endurance increases
- Energy level increases
- Weight normalizes
- Sleep improves
- Immunity increases
- Pain decreases

PSYCHOLOGICAL BENEFITS
- Somatic and kinesthetic awareness increase
- Mood improves and subjective well-being increases
- Self-acceptance and self-actualization increase
- Social adjustment increases
- Anxiety and depression decrease
- Hostility decreases

PSYCHOMOTOR FUNCTIONS IMPROVE
- Grip strength increases
- Dexterity and fine skills improve
- Eye-hand coordination improves
- Choice reaction time improves

- Steadiness improves
- Depth perception improves
- Balance improves
- Integrated functioning of body parts improves

Cognitive Function Improves
- Attention improves
- Concentration improves
- Memory improves
- Learning efficiency improves
- Symbol coding improves
- Flicker fusion frequency improves

Biochemical Effects
The biochemical profile improves, indicating an antistress and antioxidant effect, important in the prevention of degenerative diseases.

- Glucose decreases
- Sodium decreases
- Total cholesterol decreases
- Triglycerides decrease
- HDL cholesterol increases
- LDL cholesterol decreases
- VLDL cholesterol decreases
- Cholinesterase increases
- Catecholamines decrease
- ATPase increases
- Hematocrit increases
- Hemoglobin increases
- Lymphocyte count increases
- Total white blood cell count decreases
- Thyroxin increases
- Vitamin C increases
- Total serum protein increases

Yoga Compared to Conventional Exercise

Yoga	*Exercise*
Parasympathetic nervous system dominates	Sympathetic nervous system dominates
Subcortical regions of brain dominate	Cortical regions of brain dominate
Slow dynamic and static movements	Rapid, forceful movements
Normalization of muscle tone	Increased muscle tension
Low risk of injuring muscles and ligaments	Higher risk of injury
Low caloric consumption	Moderate to high caloric consumption
Effort is minimized, relaxed	Effort is maximized
Energizing (breathing is natural or controlled)	Fatiguing (breathing is taxed)
Balanced activity of opposing muscle groups	Imbalanced activity of opposing groups
Noncompetitive, process-oriented	Competitive, goal oriented
Awareness is internal (focus is on breath and the infinite)	Awareness is external (focus is on reaching the toes, reaching the finish line, etc.)
Limitless possibilities for growth in self-awareness	Boredom factor

Select General References

Anantharaman, V., and Sarada Subrahmanyam. "Physiological Benefits in Hatha Yoga Training," *The Yoga Review,* 3: pp. 9–24.

Arpita. "Physiological and Psychological Effects of Hatha Yoga: A Review of the Literature," *The Journal of the International Association of Yoga Therapists* 1 (1990): pp. 1–28.

Bhole, M. V. "Some Neuro-physiological Correlates of Yogasanas," *Yoga-Mimamsa* 19 (April 1977): pp. 53–61.

Cole, Roger. "Physiology of Yoga," *Iyengar Yoga Institute Review* (October 1985).

Corby, J. C., W. T. Roth, V. P. Zarcone, Jr., and B. S. Kopell. "Psychophysiological Correlates of the Practice of Tantric Yoga Meditation," *Archives of General Psychiatry* 35 (May 1978): pp. 571–77.

Davidson, Julian M. "The Physiology of Meditation and Mystical States of Consciousness," *Perspectives in Biology and Medicine* 19 (1976): pp. 345–79.

Delmonte, M. M. "Physiological Concomitants of Meditation Practice," *International Journal of Psychosomatics* 31 (1984): pp. 23–36.

———. "Physiological Responses During Meditation and Rest," *Biofeedback Self Regulation* 9 (January 1984): pp. 181–200.

———. "Biochemical Indices Associated with Meditation Practice: A Literature Review," *Neuroscience and Biobehavioral Reviews* 9 (Winter 1985): pp. 557–61.

Dostaleck, C. "Physiological Bases of Yoga Techniques in the Prevention of Diseases," CIANS-ISBM Satellite Conference Symposium, Hanover, Germany, 1992: Lifestyle Changes in the Prevention and Treatment of Disease. *Homeostasis in Health and Disease* 35 (1994): pp. 205–8.

Ebert, Dietrich. "Yoga from the Point of View of Psychophysiology," *Yoga-Mimamsa* 28: pp. 10–21.

Elson, Barry D., Peter Hauri, and David Cunis. "Physiological Changes in Yoga Meditation," *Psychophysiology* 14 (January 1977): pp. 52–57.

Engel, K. *Meditation.* Vol. 2. *Empirical Research and Theory.* Frankfurt, Germany: Peter Lang, 1997.

Funderburk, James. *Science Studies Yoga: A Review of Physiological Data.* Honesdale, PA.: Himalayan International Institute, 1977.

Gopal, K. S., O. P. Bhatnagar, N. Subramanian, and S. D. Nishith. *Indian Journal of Physiology and Pharmacy* 17 (1973): pp. 273–76.

Jevning, R., A. F. Wilson, and J. M. Davidson. "Adrenocortical Activity During Meditation." *Hormones & Behavior* 10: pp. 54–60. pp 2–1978.

Jevning, R., R. K. Wallace, and M. Beidebach. "The Physiology of Meditation: A Review. A Wakeful Hypometabolic Integrated Response," *Neuroscience and Biobehavioral Reviews* 16 (Fall 1992): pp. 415–24.

King, Roy, M. D., and Ann Brownstone. "Neurophysiology of Yoga Meditation," *International Journal of Yoga Therapy* 9 (1999): pp. 9–17.

Kuvalayananda, Swami. "Some Physiological Aspects of Meditative Poses," *Yoga-Mimamsa* 3 (1928): pp. 245–50.

————. "Physiology of Pranayama," *Kalyana-Kalpataru* 7 (1940) pp. 219–28.

Mager J, V. Pratap, B. Levitt, J. Hanifin, and G. Brainard. "The Influence of Classical Yoga Practices on Plasma Cortisol Levels." Poster #P3-196. The 85th Annual Meeting of the Endocrine Society, Philadelphia, PA.: (June 19–22, 2003).

Majmundar, Matra. *Physiology of Yoga Therapeutics* (working title). Forthcoming.

Malathi, A., Neela Patil, Nilesh Shah, A. Damodaran, and S. K. Marathe, "Promotive, Prophylactic Benefits of Yogic Practices in Middle-aged Women," *International Journal of Yoga Therapy,* forthcoming 2001, no. 11.

Motoyama, Hiroshi. *A Psychophysiological Study of Yoga.* Tokyo: Institute for Religious Psychology, 1976.

Murphy, M., and S. Donovan. *The Physiological and Psychological Effects of Meditation: A Review of Contemporary Research with a Comprehensive Bibliography 1931–1996.* 2d ed. Sausalito, CA: The Institute of Noetic Sciences, 1997.

Pero, G., and G. Spoto. "Study on the Anatomy of Yoga Asana and Their Neurological Effect: A Comparative Study," *Yoga-Mimamsa* 24 (1985): pp. 17–18.

Roney-Dougal, S. M. "On a Possible Psychophysiology of the Yogic Chakra System," *Journal of Indian Psychology* 17 (July 1999).

Sahu, R. J., and M. V. Bhole. "Effect of 3 Weeks Yogic Training Programme on Psycho-motor Performance," *Yoga-Mimamsa* 22 (1983): pp. 59–62.

Santha, Joseph, K. Shridharan, S. K. B. Patil, M. L. Kumaria, W. Selvamurthy, and H. S. Nayar. "Neurohumoral and Metabolic Changes Consequent to Yogic Exercises," *Indian Journal of Medical Research* 74 (1981): pp. 120–24.

————, K. Shridharan, S. K. B. Patil, M. L. Kumaria, W. Selvamurthy, N. T. Joseph, and H. S. Nayar. "Study of Some Physiological and Biochemical Parameters in Subjects Undergoing Yogic Training," *Indian Journal of Medical Research* 74 (July 1981): pp. 120–24.

Schell, F. J., B. Allolio, and O. W. Schonecke. "Physiological and Psychological Effects of Hatha-Yoga Exercise in Healthy Women," *International Journal of Psychosomatics* 41 (1994): pp. 46–52.

Selvamurthy, W., H. S. Nayar, N. T. Joseph, and S. Joseph. "Physiological Effects of Yogic Practices," *NIMHANS (National Institute of Mental Health and Neuro Sciences of India) Journal* 1 (January 1983): pp. 71–79.

Singh, R. H., R. M. Shettiwar, and K. N. Udupa. "Physiological and Therapeutic Studies on Yoga," *The Yoga Review* 2 (1982): pp. 185–209.

————, and K. N. Udupa. "Psychobiological Studies on Some Hatha-Yogic Practices," *Quarterly Journal of Surgical Sciences* 13 (1977): pp. 290–93.

Udupa, K. N., R. H. Singh, and R. M. Shettiwar. "Studies on Physiological, Endocrine, and Metabolic Responses to the Practice of 'Yoga' in Young Normal Volunteers," *Journal of Research in Indian Medicine* 6 (1971): pp. 345–53.

————. "Studies on Physiological and Metabolic Response to the Practice of

Yoga in Young Normal Volunteers," *Journal of Research in Indian Medicine* 6 (1972): pp. 345–53.

————. "Physiological and Biochemical Changes Following the Practice of Some Yogic and Non-Yogic Exercises," *Journal of Research in Indian Medicine* 10 (1975): pp. 91–93.

————. "Physiological and Biochemical Studies on the Effect of Yoga and Certain Other Exercises." *Indian Journal of Medical Research* 63 (1975): pp. 620–25.

————. "A Comparative Study on the Effect of Some Individual Yogic Practices in Normal Persons," *Indian Journal of Medical Research* 63 (1975): pp. 1960–71.

————, R. H. Singh, and R. A. Yadav. "Certain Studies on Psychological and Biochemical Responses to the Practice of Hatha Yoga in Young Normal Volunteers," *Indian Journal of Medical Research* 61 (1973): pp. 231–44.

Wallace, Robert, and H. Benson. "The Physiology of Meditation," *Scientific American* 226 (February 1972): pp. 84–90.

Wenger, M. A., and B. K. Bagchi. "Studies of Autonomic Functions in Practitioners of Yoga in India," *Behavioral Science* 6 (1961): pp. 312–23.

West, Michael A. "Physiological Effects of Meditation: A Longitudinal Study," *British Journal of Social and Clinical Psychology* 18 (June 1979): pp. 219–26.

Woolfolk, Robert L. "Psychophysiological Correlates of Meditation," *Archives of General Psychiatry* 32 (October 1975): pp. 1326–33.

Yoga: The Poses

Following are twenty-six yoga poses that provide an excellent regimen and offer all the benefits described above. Because yoga is so much more than just a workout routine, I went to Richard Rosen, a leading yoga expert for instruction on each pose. Richard is the deputy director of the Yoga Research and Education Center (www.yrec.org), headed by Georg Feuerstein. Richard is a contributing editor at *Yoga Journal,* for which he writes two regular columns as well as book reviews and articles. His work has also appeared in *Yoga International, Ascent,* and *Yoga Aktuell,* the national German yoga magazine. He is the author of *The Yoga of Breath,* a beginners' guide to *pranayama.* Richard has been teaching yoga since 1987.

1. EASY POSE (*Sukhasana*)

Sit on the floor and cross your legs at the shins. Lay your hands in your lap (as shown in the illustration), or rest them on your knees, palms down. If you tend to slump backward when sitting flat on the floor in Easy Pose or if your back starts to ache, sit on a firm pillow or thick, folded blanket. You should be able to sit so that your hipbones are relatively parallel to the floor. This will ensure that your spine is properly lengthened. Lift your chest, relax your shoulders away from your ears, and lightly balance your head atop your spine. If you practice this pose regularly, be sure to alternate how you cross your shins: right leg forward one day (as shown here), left leg forward the next.

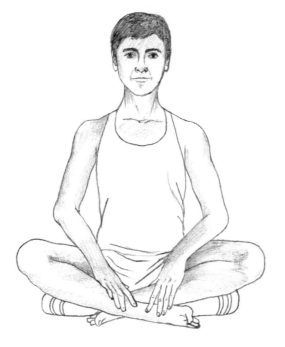

2. PERFECT POSE (*Siddhasana*)

This sitting pose is a more challenging version of Easy Pose. Sit on the floor with your legs extended in front of you. Bend your right knee and draw the heel close to, but not touching, your groin, and then let the knee and shin drop as close to the floor as you can. Next, bend your left knee and tuck the left foot between your right calf and thigh. Release but don't force your left knee toward the floor. If the left knee is above the floor, support it with a thickly folded blanket or thick book.

Bring the right heel completely into the groin, tucking the right foot between the left calf and thigh. Sit so your hipbones are relatively parallel to the floor. If you can't, and you tend to slump, be sure to sit on either a firm pillow or folded blanket. Lift your chest, relax your shoulders away from your ears, and lightly balance your head atop your spine. Lay your hands on your knees, either palms up (as shown in the illustration) or, if your shoulders are tight, palms down. Remember that if you practice this pose regularly, be sure to alternate how you cross your legs: left leg on top one day, right leg on top the next.

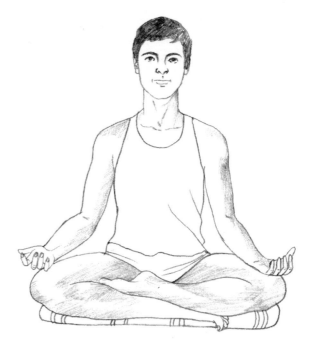

3. MOUNTAIN POSE (*Tadasana*)

Stand with your feet parallel, a few inches apart. Firm your thighs and turn them slightly in but keep your belly soft. Draw your pubic bone gently up, toward your navel, and imagine that your tailbone is lengthening downward toward the floor. Lift and widen your chest and relax your shoulders away from your ears. Hold your head lightly on the top of your spine so that your chin is parallel to the floor. Press your palms firmly together in front of your torso, either at the level of the belly or higher, in front of your heart (as shown in the illustration).

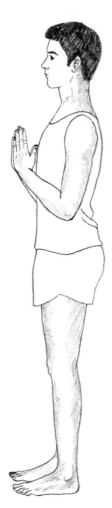

4. RAISED-ARMS MOUNTAIN POSE
(*Urdhyá Hastá Tadasana*)

From Mountain Pose 4, inhale and lift your arms overhead. Join your palms only if you can keep your shoulders soft and neck long and relaxed; if your shoulders and neck tense when the palms are joined, keep your arms apart, parallel to each other. Make sure, when raising your arms, that you don't arch your lower back. Keep the lower back long by continuing to lift your pubis and lengthen your tailbone. Keep your chin parallel to the floor. Stretch toward the ceiling through your fingertips, pressing the thumbs against or angling them away from the index fingers (as shown in the illustration). Exhale and lower your arms to your sides.

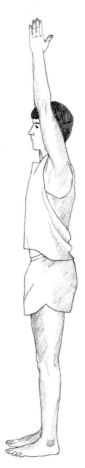

SUN SALUTATION (*Surya Namaskar*)

5. STANDING FORWARD BEND
   (*Uttanasana,* literally "intense stretch pose")

From Raised-Arms Mountain Pose 4, exhale, sweep your arms out to the sides, and bend forward. Make sure you bend from your hip, not your waist, so that you keep your front torso long. Release your hands to the floor (as shown in the illustration). If your hands don't reach the floor, cross your forearms and hold your elbows. Don't struggle to touch the floor. Firm your thighs. If the backs of your thighs or your lower back feel uncomfortable, bend your knees slightly.

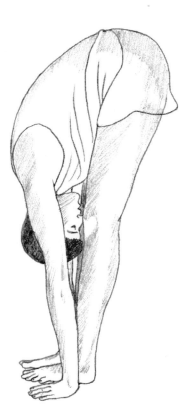

6. LEFT LUNGE (*Anjaneyasana*)

From Standing Forward Bend, Pose 5, inhale, shift your weight onto your left foot. Bend your left knee as you slowly step back three to four feet with your right foot. Bend your right knee to the floor. If you're practicing on an uncarpeted floor, you might want to kneel on a folded blanket. Align your left knee directly over your left ankle, and slide your right knee back along the floor until you feel a comfortable stretch in the thigh and front groin. As you do this, roll the right hip slightly forward to keep the pelvis facing front as much as possible. Press your fingertips against the floor (as shown in the illustration) and lift your chest. Look straight ahead.

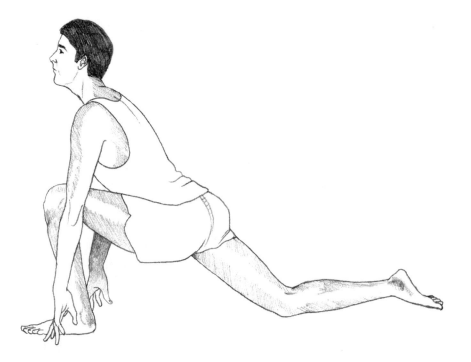

7. DOWNWARD FACING DOG
(*Adho Mukha Svanasana*)

From the Bent-Knee Lunge, exhale, press your palms firmly against the floor, and step back with your left foot, placing it beside the right. At the same time, lift your pelvis up and back. Separate your hands and feet, strengthen your arms and legs, and stretch your heels toward the floor. Strengthen your legs by firming the front thighs, but be sure not to lock your knees. Align your head between your arms, and draw your shoulders away from your ears.

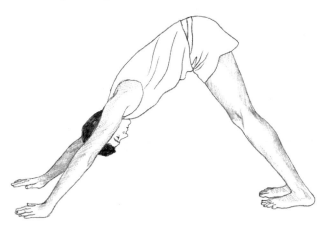

8. PLANK POSE (*Chaturanga Dandasana*)

From Downward Facing Dog inhale and swing your torso down, as shown in the illustration.

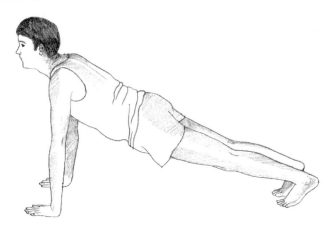

9. COBRA POSE (*Bhujangasana*)

From Plank Pose, exhale, bend your elbows, and lower your torso and legs toward the floor. Inhale, then quickly straighten your arms and raise your chest up and forward. Position your shoulders, if possible, directly over your wrists, and relax your shoulders away from your ears. Strengthen your legs, firm your buttocks, and press your tailbone down, toward your pubis. Your legs can rest on the floor (as shown in the illustration). If your legs are slightly off the floor, with only the tops of your feet pressing down, the pose is called Upward Facing Dog (*urdhva mukha svanasana*). Be careful not to jam your lower back. Look straight ahead or, without squeezing the back of your neck, drop your head back and gaze upward.

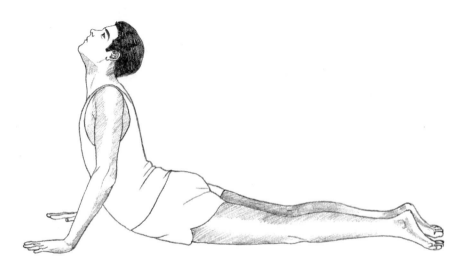

10. DOWNWARD FACING DOG
(*Adho Mukha Shvanasana*)
From Cobra Pose exhale and push up into Downward Facing Dog.

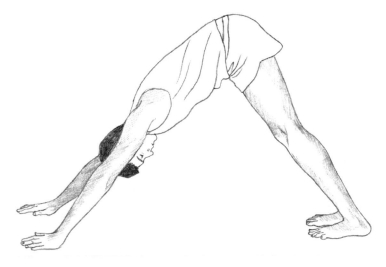

11. RIGHT LUNGE (*Anjaneyasana*)
From Downward Facing Dog inhale. Step forward on your right foot to lunge. Keep your back leg strong and straight. Lift the front of the left thigh away from the floor and press actively through the left heel. Lay the weight of your torso on the top of the right thigh.

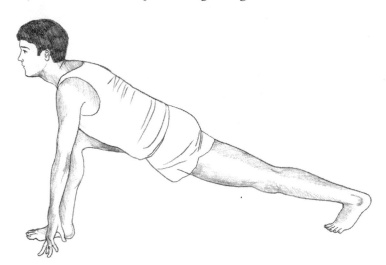

12. STANDING FORWARD BEND (*Uttanasana*)

From Right Lunge exhale and bring your left foot beside the right.

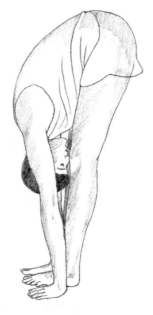

13. RAISED-ARMS MOUNTAIN POSE
(*Urdhva Hasta Tadasana*)

From Standing Forward Bend inhale and sweep your arms out to the sides and then overhead. Join your palms or keep your hands separate but parallel. Keep the ribs down and lengthen your tailbone. Stretch your arms toward the ceiling.

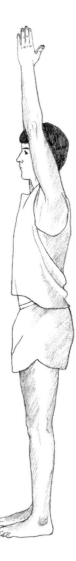

14. MOUNTAIN POSE (*Tadasana*)

Exhale and lower the arms. Clasp your hands in front of your heart or belly. Repeat the entire sequence, but do a right lunge first. This will complete one full cycle of Sun Salutation. Perform from three to ten full cycles.

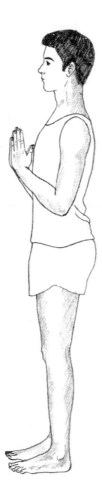

NOTE: For all the sitting poses following (including 16, 23, 24), if you tend to slump backward when sitting flat on the floor, or if your un-supported back starts to ache, be sure to sit on a firm pillow or thickly folded blanket.

15. SITTING BENT-KNEE FORWARD BEND
(*Janu Sirsasana,* literally "head-to-knee pose")

Sit on the floor with your legs extended in front of you. Bend your left knee and draw the heel into the groin. Let the left knee and thigh relax toward the floor. Keep the left sole to the side of the right thigh; don't allow it to slide underneath the thigh.

Turn your torso slightly to the right, to face over your right leg, and reach for the sides of your right foot. Press actively through your right heel. If you can't stretch far enough to touch your right foot or if you can do it only by rounding forward and hunching your back, wrap a cloth strap or belt around the right sole, and hold the strap in both hands. Start out with your arms fully extended and the front of your torso lifted and long. Exhale and lower into the forward bend. Be sure not to use the strap to pull yourself into the pose. Keep your arms long and gently walk your hands along the strap as far as you can. Stop when the front of your torso begins to round and shorten. If you're holding your foot, simply bend your elbows out to the sides as you fold forward.

Hold the pose anywhere from one to three minutes. Then inhale and lift your torso. Repeat with the left leg forward.

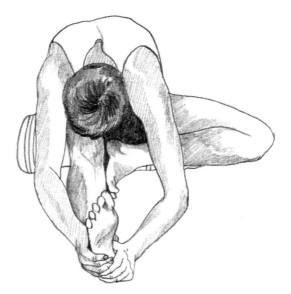

16. YOGA CURL-UP

Lie on your back, your knees bent, feet on the floor. Clasp your hands at the back of your head. Lay your arms on the floor, elbows down. Exhale and curl your torso up, twisting slightly to the left. At the same time, lift your left knee toward your torso. Now aim your right elbow toward the raised left knee, hold, and inhale. Then exhale and roll your torso back to the floor as you put your left foot beside the right foot. Repeat, raising the right knee and using the left elbow. Be sure not to pull your torso up by using your arms. Use your abdominal muscles to create the lift. Repeat five to eight times with each leg at first, then gradually build up the number of repetitions over time.

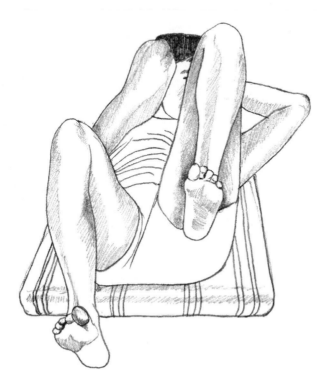

17. WARRIOR POSE (*Virabhadrasana III.* Named after the Indian warrior Virabhadra, this pose is considered the third of three Warrior Pose variations)

Stand in Raised-Arms Mountain Pose, 13. Inhale and shift your weight onto your right foot. Exhale, strengthen your left leg, and raise the left leg as you lower your torso and arms. Position the torso, arms, and the raised leg parallel to the floor, as much as you can. The left hip tends to lift a little higher than the right hip, so roll the left hip slightly down until the front of your pelvis is about parallel to the floor. Align your head between your arms (as shown in the illustration) or lift it slightly and gaze forward.

If you find yourself toppling over, use a wall for support until your balance is better. First face the wall with your hands pressed against it at about hip height; step back until your arms and torso are parallel to the floor and your heels are directly below your hips, so that your legs are perpendicular to the floor. Push off the wall, inhale, and lift your arms to Raised-Arms Mountain Pose. Then exhale and bind forward into the pose, hands touching the wall. Use the wall to steady yourself and maintain your balance. Don't lean on it.

Hold this pose anywhere from thirty seconds to one minute. Inhale and return to Raised-Arms Mountain Pose. Lower your arms for a few seconds, and then repeat for the same length of time standing on your left foot.

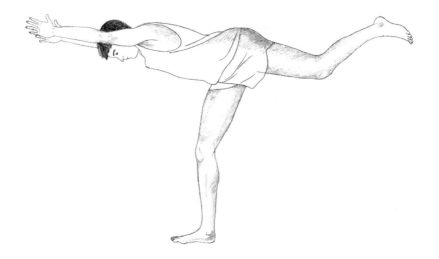

18. TREE POSE (*Vrksasana*)

Stand in Mountain Pose, 14. Inhale, shift your weight onto your left foot and lift your right foot off the floor. Reach down with your right hand, grip your right ankle, and draw the sole up onto your inner left knee. If your hips are flexible, you can position the right foot at the top of the thigh. Press your palms together in front of your heart. Gaze steadily at an imaginary point about four feet in front of you on the floor.

If you find yourself toppling over, use a wall for support until your balance is better. Stand with your back resting on the wall, with your heels a couple of inches away from it. Move into the pose as described. After a few breaths, press your hands against the wall beside your hips, and lift your torso free of the wall. As you hold the pose, gradually reduce the pressure of your hands on the wall, until they leave the wall entirely and you're balancing unsupported. Then press the hands together in front of your heart.

Hold this pose for thirty seconds to one minute, exhale, and lower the right foot back to the floor. Repeat, raising the left foot.

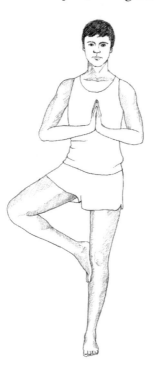

19 and 20. CAT POSE (*Marjariasana*)

Start on all fours, knees beneath the hips, hands beneath the shoulders. Inhale, arch your back, and lift your head to look up. Then exhale, round your back, and press (but don't force) your chin toward your chest. Be sure to engage your entire spine as you move, especially the area between the shoulder blades. Repeat slowly five to ten times, moving in rhythm with your breathing.

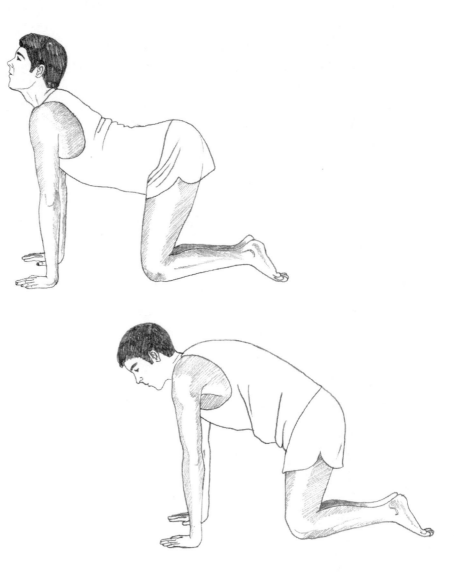

21. UPWARD BOW (*Urdhva Dhanurasana*)
(Sometimes called the Wheel)

Lie on your back with your knees bent, feet on the floor, heels near your buttocks, toes turned in. Place your palms on the floor at either side of your head, fingers turned toward your shoulders. Inhale, arch your torso away from the floor, and rest the crown of your head on the floor. Take a few breaths, make sure your arms and especially the legs are perpendicular to the floor. Then exhale and push yourself up into the full back bend.

Keep your feet and thighs parallel. Turn your upper thighs slightly inward, firm your tailbone against the back of the pelvis, and lift your pubis toward your navel. Let your head hang or lift it slightly and look at the floor (as shown in the illustration).

Hold the pose anywhere from five to ten seconds, breathing easily. Exhale and return to lying on the floor. Repeat from three to five times. Then draw your thighs up to your torso, clasp your arms around your legs, hugging them to your chest.

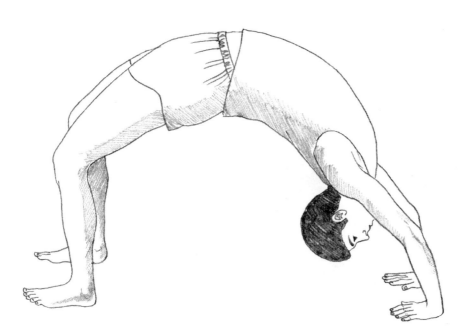

22. SITTING FORWARD BEND (*Paschimottanasana,* literally "intense-stretch-of-the west Pose," the "west" being the back of the body)

Sit on the floor with your legs extended in front of you. Firm your thighs and press actively through your heels. Lean forward slightly and grip the outside edges of your feet. If you can't reach your feet or can do so only by rounding forward and hunching your back, wrap a cloth or belt around your feet and hold the strap in both hands. Start out with your arms fully extended and the front of your torso lifted and long. Exhale and lower into the forward bend. Be sure not to use the strap to pull yourself into the pose. Instead, keep your arms long and gently walk your hands along the strap as far as you can. Stop when the front of your torso begins to round and shorten. If you're holding your feet, simply bend your elbows out to the sides as you fold forward.

Hold the pose anywhere from one to three minutes, then inhale and lift your torso.

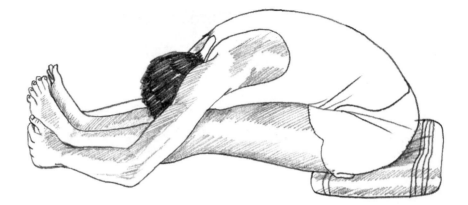

23. HALF KING OF THE FISH POSE
(*Ardha Matsyendrasana*)

Sit on the floor with your legs extended in front of you. Then bend your knees and draw your feet up on the floor to about a foot away from your pelvis. Slide your left heel to the outside of your right hip and lay the left thigh on the floor. Then cross your right leg over the left, bringing your right foot to the outside of your left thigh with the sole of the foot on the floor. Tuck your right heel as close as you can to your left hip, and press the foot actively against the floor.

Inhale and lift your chest. Then exhale and turn your torso to the right. Bring the left arm to the outside of the right thigh (as shown in the illustration), only if you can do it without rounding your torso over the leg. Otherwise, wrap your left arm around the leg and hug the inner thigh against your torso. You can turn your head to the right (as shown in the illustration) or look over your left shoulder, down at your right foot.

Hold the pose for a minute. Lift the torso with each inhalation, twisting a little more with each exhalation. Exhale, uncross the legs, then recross with the left over right. Hold for the same length of time.

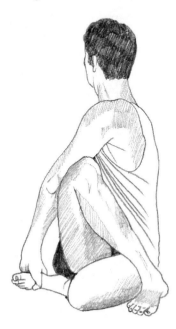

24. LOCUST PREPARATION POSE

This is a preparation for the next pose, Locust. Lie facedown. If you're practicing on an uncarpeted floor, lie on a mat or a folded blanket. Place your arms at your sides, palms up. Firm your buttocks and press your tailbone down, toward the pubis. Inhale, lift your legs a few inches off the floor, hold for a few seconds, then exhale and place legs back on floor.

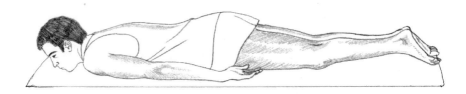

25. LOCUST (*Salabhasana*)

From Locust Preparation Pose, inhale and lift your legs, arms, upper torso, and head. Turn the big toes toward each other, so your legs are rolled slightly inward. Keep your lower ribs and pelvis on the floor. Raise your arms parallel to the floor, relax your shoulders away from your ears, and reach back through the arms and legs as you open your sternum forward. Lift your head a bit and gaze forward.

Hold the pose anywhere from thirty seconds to one minute. Exhale and release. Then repeat once or twice more.

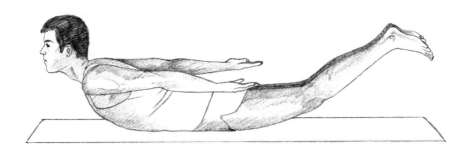

26. COBRA POSE (*Bhujangasana*)

Lie on your belly, arms extended forward along the floor, palms down. Strengthen your legs, firm your buttocks, and press your tailbone down, toward your pubis. Lift your upper torso and head, bend your elbows, and slide your forearms back until your elbows are positioned directly below your shoulders (so the upper arms are perpendicular to the floor). Hold for a few breaths, feeling the stretch in your belly. Then slowly move your forearms away from the floor until the elbows are straight. Be careful not to jam your lower back. If your lower back feels relatively comfortable, walk your hands gradually back underneath (or nearly underneath) your shoulders. Look straight forward or, without squeezing the back of your neck, drop your head back and gaze upward. Hold for thirty seconds to one minute, breathing easily, then release to lie fully stretched on the floor. Repeat once or twice more.

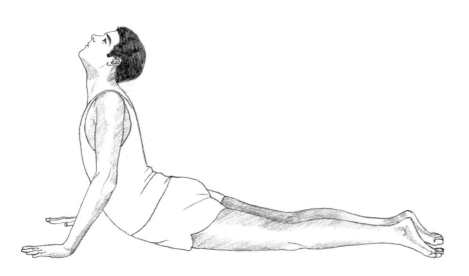

8

Dr. Perricone's 28-Day Acne-Free Program

An integral part of my total-body acne-fighting program is my 28-day diet. Health and good looks begin on the inside. The 28-Day Program is simple, nutritious, and, best of all, delicious. A number of the recipes were created exclusively for the Perricone Program by award-winning executive chef Bernard Guillas. See Appendix A for the recipes of these mouthwatering dishes you can prepare in your own kitchen.

Important Tips

- Eat protein first! Always remember to start your meal with protein. It may seem odd to eat fish before soup, but doing so will ensure that you avoid a glycemic response.
- Eat salmon. Salmon is a major component of both the three-day and the 28-day plans. The reason is simple. Salmon is extremely high in protein and essential fatty acids. Salmon also contains DMAE, which increases skin health, tone, and radiance.
- Get enough essential fatty acids. Omega-3 essential fatty acids are an important component in the treatment and prevention of acne. In addition to eating plenty of coldwater fish—such as salmon, sardines, anchovies, and so on—add flaxseed to your diet as another high-quality source of the omega-3s. Flaxseed can be purchased in any natural food store and should be stored in the freezer. Buy a

small food grinder (such as those used for grinding coffee beans or nuts) and grind a cup at a time to store in the freezer. You will always have some on hand to sprinkle on oatmeal, yogurt, berries, and so forth to impart a delicious, nutty flavor.

- Feel free to mix and match—the suggested meals are to be used as a guideline. All of Chef Bernard's recipes are a gourmet treat and great for the skin. Most of the recipes serve six. When I suggest 4 to 6 ounces of chicken or fish, that is for an individual serving.

- Think green! Eat plenty of vegetables such as garlic, onions, broccoli, and dark greens. Fresh herbs, such as oregano, are also rich in antioxidants.

- Be sure to include foods, such as whole yogurt, that contain probiotics which are very beneficial for the treatment of acne.

- Try PomWonderful pomegranate juice. These slightly tart, delicious fruit juices are very high in antioxidants.

- Although I have included a number of delightful gourmet recipes, please also remember that 4 to 6 ounces of baked, grilled, or broiled fish or chicken breast lightly brushed with olive oil makes a simple lunch or dinner. Add a tossed dark-green leafy salad dressed with olive oil and lemon juice, a vegetable from the list of good carbohydrates, and you have a healthy meal with a minimum of time and effort.

- Buy organic eggs from free-range hens at the natural food store or the health food department of your supermarket; there you will be more likely to find eggs that are very high in the omega-3 essential fatty acids.

- For salad dressings and marinades I recommend extra virgin olive oil and the fresh lemon juice. Adjust to taste.

- When possible use fresh herbs for their superior flavor and antioxidants.

- In this chapter we present menu plans for 14 days. At the end of the 14 days go back to day one and repeat to complete the 28-Day-Program.

- When baking or grilling fish or poultry, first brush lightly with olive oil.

- Feel free to substitute tofu or tempeh for fish or chicken. However, if possible try to eat Alaskan salmon in some form (canned, frozen, or fresh) at least three times a week for its incomparable benefits to your skin.
- Instead of rice use pearled or whole barley, or whole oats. They can also be used in risotto recipes, soups, stir-fries, and in any dish in which you would normally use rice or other grains.
- Drink green tea, a refreshing beverage whether hot or iced. Add fresh lemon juice for both flavor and antioxidants. Research has shown that green tea contains compounds that help the body metabolize fat as well as encourage feelings of well-being.
- Take your supplements twice a day with water, preferably at mealtimes.
- Make exercise an integral part of your daily routine. I have indicated that you exercise first thing in the morning; I find physical activity to be a wonderful way to start the day. But feel free to take ten or fifteen minutes at other times during the day—whenever you feel a need to destress and/or reinvigorate yourself.

Note: Recipes for dishes marked with an asterisk appear in Appendix A.

WATER =

YOGA =

SUPPLEMENTS =

TOPICALS =

Week One
Day 1: Monday
Wake up with an 8-ounce glass of water

Yoga

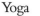
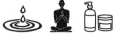

BREAKFAST
- 3 to 4 ounces smoked Nova Scotia salmon
- ½ cup slow-cooked oatmeal
- 1 teaspoon slivered almonds
- 8 ounces green tea or water

LUNCH
- 4- to 6-ounce grilled turkey burger (no bun)
- Lettuce and a tomato slice
- ½ cup three-bean salad (chickpeas, kidney, and black beans dressed with olive oil, fresh lemon juice to taste, and a minced clove of garlic) served on a bed of cabbage leaves
- 8 ounces water

SNACK
- 6 ounces unflavored yogurt mixed with 1 tablespoon PomWonderful pomegranate juice
- 8 ounces water

DINNER
- 1 cup lentil soup
- Spiced Diver Scallops★
- Green salad dressed with olive oil and fresh lemon juice to taste
- 2-inch wedge of cantaloupe
- 8 ounces water

BEDTIME
- 1 hard-boiled egg
- 2 celery sticks
- 3 Brazil nuts
- 8 ounces water

Day 2: Tuesday
Wake up with an 8-ounce glass of water

Yoga

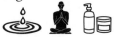

BREAKFAST
- 2-egg omelet
- Sliced tomato
- ½ cup blueberries topped with 3 chopped almonds
- 8 ounces green tea or water

LUNCH
- 3 to 6 ounces grilled salmon or one small (3 to 4 ounces) can of salmon
- Green salad (1 cup romaine lettuce, one small sliced tomato, sliced cucumber, diced red onion, and 2 tablespoons chickpeas) dressed with olive oil, fresh lemon juice to taste, and a minced clove of garlic
- 1 small apple
- 8 ounces water

SNACK
- ½ cup cottage cheese sprinkled with 1 tablespoon ground flaxseed
- 2 pears
- 8 ounces water

DINNER

- Feta and Spinach–Stuffed Chicken Breast with Warm Green Bean and Pear Salad and Grilled Heirloom Tomatoes★
- Ecuadorian Tabouleh★
- Romaine lettuce salad dressed with olive oil and fresh lemon juice to taste
- 8 ounces water

BEDTIME

- 2 ounces sliced roast turkey breast
- ¼ cup pumpkin seeds
- 2-inch wedge of honeydew melon
- 8 ounces water

Day 3: Wednesday

Wake up with an 8-ounce glass of water
Yoga

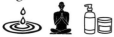

BREAKFAST

- 2 slices turkey bacon
- 1 poached or over-easy egg
- ½ cup strawberries
- 3 almonds
- 8 ounces green tea or water

LUNCH

- 3- to 4-ounce can of tuna, shrimp, or salmon
- Tomato and cucumber slices
- ½ cup three-bean salad (chickpeas, kidney, and black beans

dressed with olive oil, fresh lemon juice to taste, and a minced clove of garlic)
- 8 ounces water

SNACK
- 6 ounces unflavored yogurt mixed with 1 tablespoon PomWonderful pomegranate juice
- 3 Brazil nuts
- 8 ounces water

DINNER
- Smoked Salmon Rillette★ or 4 to 6 ounces grilled or baked salmon
- 6 spears steamed asparagus
- Butter Lettuce, Radish, and Hearts of Palm Salad★
- 2-inch wedge of cantaloupe
- 8 ounces water

BEDTIME
- 2 ounces sliced chicken or turkey breast
- 4 almonds
- 1 apple or pear
- 8 ounces water

Day 4: Thursday

Wake up with an 8-ounce glass of water

Yoga

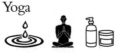

BREAKFAST
- ½ cup slow-cooked oatmeal topped with 1 tablespoon ground flaxseed or chopped pumpkin seeds
- 2 turkey sausage links

- ½ cup blueberries
- 8 ounces green tea or water

Lunch
- 4 ounces grilled or baked chicken diced and mixed with fresh dill, chopped red onion, garlic, olive oil, and lemon juice and garnished with 3 chopped almonds
- ½ cup steamed broccoli
- ½ cup mixed berries (strawberries, blueberries, raspberries)
- 8 ounces water

Snack
- 2 slices roast turkey breast
- 4 cherry tomatoes
- 3 Brazil nuts
- 8 ounces water

Dinner
- Tofu Vegetable Stir-fry★ (substitute chicken or turkey if you prefer)
- 2-inch wedge of cantaloupe
- 8 ounces water

Bedtime
- 6 ounces unflavored yogurt mixed with 1 tablespoon PomWonderful pomegranate juice
- 3 almonds or hazelnuts
- 8 ounces water

Day 5: Friday

Wake up with an 8-ounce glass of water

Yoga

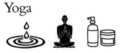

BREAKFAST

- 2 slices turkey bacon
- ½ cup slow-cooked oatmeal seasoned with cinnamon
- 2 teaspoons chopped almonds
- 2-inch wedge of cantaloupe
- 8 ounces green tea or water

LUNCH

- 4 ounces finely cubed salmon filet or canned salmon dressed with olive oil, fresh lemon juice to taste, and fresh dill and served on bed of romaine lettuce
- ½ cup lentil soup
- 8 ounces water or green tea

SNACK

- 2 slices turkey
- ½ cup berries
- 4 almonds or Brazil nuts
- 8 ounces water

DINNER

- Pan-Seared Organic Sonoma Chicken Breast★
- Wilted Leeks and Swiss Chard★
- ½ cup three-bean salad (white, black, and pinto beans or lentils marinated in olive oil and fresh lemon juice to taste)
- 8 ounces water

BEDTIME
- 6 ounces unflavored yogurt mixed with 1 tablespoon PomWonderful™ pomegranate juice
- 4 walnuts
- 8 ounces water

Day 6: Saturday
Wake up with an 8-ounce glass of water
Yoga

BREAKFAST
- 2-egg omelet filled with ½ cup mushrooms and spinach
- 1 slice Canadian or turkey bacon
- 2-inch wedge of honeydew melon
- 8 ounces green tea or water

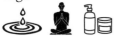

LUNCH
- 4 to 6 ounces broiled salmon
- 1 cup Caesar salad without croutons (romaine lettuce tossed with 1 clove minced garlic, olive oil, and lemon juice; top with 1 tablespoon grated cheese such as pecorino Romano)
- 1 apple
- 8 ounces water

SNACK
- 6 ounces unflavored yogurt
- ½ cup mixed berries
- 3 almonds
- 8 ounces water

DINNER
- Pistachio Almond–Crusted Wild Striped Bass★
- 6 spears steamed asparagus
- ½ cup three-bean salad (white, black, and pinto beans or lentils marinated in olive oil and fresh lemon juice to taste)
- 2-inch wedge of cantaloupe

BEDTIME
- 2 slices roast turkey or chicken breast
- ¼ cup pumpkin seeds
- ½ cup cherries
- 8 ounces water

Day 7: Sunday
Wake up with an 8-ounce glass of water

Relaxation

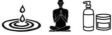

BREAKFAST
- 3 to 6 ounces broiled salmon
- ½ cup slow-cooked oatmeal
- 2-inch wedge of cantaloupe
- 8 ounces green tea or water

LUNCH
- 6-ounce can of crabmeat mixed with 1 chopped scallion and 1 chopped celery rib, dressed with ¼ cup unflavored yogurt, juice of ½ lemon served in an avocado half
- ½ cup berries (blueberries, raspberries, strawberries)
- 8 ounces water

SNACK
- ½ cup cottage cheese topped with 1 tablespoon ground flaxseed or ¼ cup chopped pumpkin seeds
- 1 apple
- 8 ounces water

DINNER
- Pomegranate–Citrus Glazed Apricot- and Garlic-Roasted Chicken with Apple-Spinach Stuffing and Garden Vegetables
- 1 kiwi
- 8 ounces water

BEDTIME
- 2 slices turkey breast
- 4 walnuts
- 1 pear
- 8 ounces water

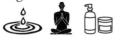

Week Two

Day 8: Monday
Wake up with an 8-ounce glass of water

Yoga

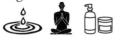

BREAKFAST
- 2 slices Canadian or turkey bacon
- ½ cup slow-cooked oatmeal topped with 1 tablespoon ground flaxseed or 2 tablespoons chopped pumpkin seeds
- ½ cup mixed berries (blueberries, raspberries, blackberries)
- 8 ounces green tea or water

LUNCH
- Greek salad (romaine lettuce, 3 black olives, 1 ounce feta, ½ sliced cucumber, 4 cherry tomatoes) dressed with olive oil, fresh lemon juice to taste, and a dash of oregano
- ½ cup of lentil soup
- 8 ounces water

SNACK
- 6 ounces unflavored yogurt mixed with 1 tablespoon PomWonderful pomegranate juice
- 3 Brazil nuts
- 8 ounces water

DINNER
- Turkey Sausage–Stuffed Portobello Mushrooms★
- Red Grape–Apple Chutney★
- 2-inch wedge of cantaloupe
- 8 ounces water

BEDTIME
- 2 ounces sliced turkey or chicken breast
- 4 almonds
- 8 ounces water

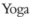

Day 9: Tuesday
Wake up with an 8-ounce glass of water.
Yoga

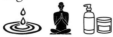

BREAKFAST:
- 2-egg omelet filled with ½ cup sautéed onions and mushrooms
- ½ cup slow-cooked oatmeal topped with 1 tablespoon ground flaxseed or 3 walnut halves
- 8 ounces green tea or water

LUNCH
- 6-ounce grilled turkey burger
- ½ cup three-bean salad (white, black, and pinto beans or lentils marinated in olive oil and fresh lemon juice to taste)
- 8 ounces water

SNACK
- 6 ounces unflavored yogurt mixed with 1 tablespoon PomWonderful pomegranate extract
- ¼ cup pumpkin seeds
- 1 apple
- 8 ounces water

DINNER
- Wild King Salmon and Tuna Sashimi with Exotic Fruit Relish★ or 6 ounces grilled salmon
- Romaine lettuce salad dressed with olive oil and fresh lemon juice to taste
- ½ cup berries (blueberries, blackberries, raspberries, strawberries)
- 8 ounces water

BEDTIME
- ½ cup cottage cheese
- ½ cup cherries
- 4 macadamia nuts
- 8 ounces water

Day 10: Wednesday

Wake up with an 8-ounce glass of water

Yoga

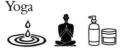

BREAKFAST

- 2 slices turkey bacon
- 2 poached or over-easy eggs
- ½ cup blueberries
- 3 Brazil nuts
- 8 ounces green tea or water

LUNCH

- 4 to 6 ounces grilled chicken
- Large green salad with sliced tomatoes and ¼ cup chickpeas
- 2-inch wedge of cantaloupe
- 8 ounces water

SNACK

- 6 ounces unflavored yogurt mixed with 1 tablespoon PomWonderful pomegranate juice
- 8 ounces water
- 3 almonds

DINNER

- Summer Gazpacho★
- Jumbo Bay Shrimp and Crabmeat Salad★
- 1 sliced kiwi
- 8 ounces water

BEDTIME
- 2 slices chicken or turkey breast
- ¼ cup pumpkin seeds
- 1 apple
- 8 ounces water

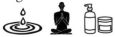

Day 11: Thursday
Wake up with an 8-ounce glass of water

Yoga

BREAKFAST
- 4 ounces smoked Nova Scotia salmon
- ½ cup slow-cooked oatmeal topped with 1 tablespoon ground flaxseed or chopped pumpkin seeds
- ¼ cup blueberries
- 8 ounces green tea or water

LUNCH
- 6-ounce can shrimp or crabmeat dressed with 1 tablespoon mayonnaise and ½ teaspoon dill, served in an avocado half
- ½ cup lentil soup
- 8 ounces water

SNACK
- 1 hard-boiled egg
- 4 cherry tomatoes
- 4 macadamia nuts
- 8 ounces water

DINNER

- East-West Chicken Breast★
- Green-Curry Barley Casserole with Green Beans★
- 1 pear
- 8 ounces water

BEDTIME

- 6 ounces unflavored yogurt mixed with 1 tablespoon PomWonderful pomegranate juice
- ½ cup blueberries
- 4 almonds
- 8 ounces water

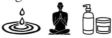

Day 12: Friday

Wake up with an 8-ounce glass of water

Yoga

BREAKFAST

- 2 eggs scrambled with chopped and sauteed onion and green or red bell peppers
- 2 slices turkey bacon
- 2-inch wedge of cantaloupe
- 8 ounces green tea or water

LUNCH

- 3 to 5 ounces cubed chicken mixed with chopped red onion and celery, dressed with olive oil and fresh lemon juice to taste, served inside an avocado half and topped with 2 tablespoons marinated chickpeas
- 8 ounces water

SNACK
- 6 ounces unflavored yogurt mixed with 1 tablespoon PomWon-derful pomegranate juice
- 4 almonds
- 8 ounces water

DINNER
- 6 ounces grilled salmon
- Romaine lettuce, and tomato salad dressed with olive oil and fresh lemon juice to taste
- Grilled zucchini and mushroom kebobs
- 8 ounces water or green tea

BEDTIME
- 2 ounces sliced turkey or chicken breast
- 4 almonds
- 1 apple
- 8 ounces water

Day 13: Saturday
Wake up with an 8-ounce glass of water
Yoga

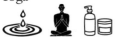

BREAKFAST
- 2 to 4 ounces smoked Nova Scotia salmon
- ½ cup unflavored yogurt
- 1 tablespoon chopped walnuts
- ½ cup blueberries
- 8 ounces green tea or water

LUNCH
- 4 to 6 ounces grilled chicken breast
- Romaine lettuce salad tossed with ½ cup white or navy beans
- 1 pear
- 8 ounces water

SNACK
- 1 hard-boiled egg
- 2-inch wedge of cantaloupe
- 4 macadamia nuts
- 8 ounces water

DINNER
- Southwestern Spiced Bluefish★
- Chickpea and Hearts of Palm Salad★
- 8 ounces water

BEDTIME
- 2 slices turkey breast
- 4 green olives
- 4 cherry tomatoes
- 8 ounces water

Day 14: Sunday

Wake up with an 8-ounce glass of water

Relaxation

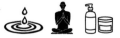

BREAKFAST
- 2-egg omelet with ½ cup sauteed mushrooms
- ½ cup slow-cooked oatmeal topped with 1 tablespoon ground flaxseed

- 2-inch wedge of cantaloupe
- 8 ounces green tea or water

LUNCH
- Romaine lettuce tossed with 3 to 4 ounces of canned tuna, ½ cup white beans, ¼ cup crumbled feta, 4 cherry tomatoes, and sliced red onion dressed with olive oil and fresh lemon juice to taste
- 8 ounces water

SNACK
- 6 ounces unflavored yogurt mixed with 1 tablespoon PomWonderful pomegranate juice
- 4 hazelnuts
- 8 ounces water

DINNER
- Mediterranean Chicken Breast with Aromatic Kidney Beans★
- ½ cup cherries
- 8 ounces water

BEDTIME
- ½ cup cottage cheese
- 4 almonds
- 1 pear
- 8 ounces water

9

The Acne-Free Future

I think the most important and exciting discovery that I ever made as a dermatologist was learning that inflammation is at the root of disease. This seemingly simple concept has revolutionized my methodology in devising effective therapies to treat inflammatory-based diseases—from acne to aging and everything in between.

And so, when we contemplate what the future may hold in developing new therapies for treating and preventing acne, we now know that the foundation of these therapies must be anti-inflammatories. In my opinion, anti-inflammatories are not confined to one specific therapeutic agent. I am speaking of the entire spectrum—a completely holistic approach that consists of placing the body in an overall anti-inflammatory state so that its susceptibility to disease is greatly diminished. This means, as Perricone readers know, following the anti-inflammatory lifestyle of:

- Eating an anti-inflammatory diet
- Taking supplements with anti-inflammatory activity
- Applying topical anti-inflammatories
- Maintaining low levels of stress
- Practicing a regular exercise routine in moderation

In addition, new delivery systems are extremely exciting. For example, the transdermal delivery of glutathione represents an important step in helping us to maintain adequate levels of this critical tripeptide. Adequate levels of glutathione are absolutely necessary to treat and prevent diseases of all types.

All too often traditional therapies are designed to treat a specific condition without looking at the overall person affected by the condition. Often these therapies fail because they do not address the underlying condition of which the disease is just a symptom. When it comes to acne, this means that while there may be an initial clearing of breakouts, the acne lesions will eventually return if the underlying cause has not been treated.

The body is incredibly complex—composed of trillions of cells that make up our vital organs. At one time the prevailing wisdom held that some master organ (for example, the endocrine system or the brain) was responsible for most communication with the cells. The reality is not that simple. We now know that there is an elaborate messenger system above and beyond hormones and nerve impulses. When cells talk to other cells, messengers within the cells control all functions, from energy production to control of the DNA.

Inflammation can be created or controlled by this highly structured intercellular messenger system, and the treatment options of the future for aging and age-related diseases (as well as other inflammatory diseases, such as acne) will revolve around understanding and controlling the information system of the cells. These messengers, some of which are called transcription factors, and the tiny strings of amino acids known as peptides and cytokines, will be the "magic bullets" dreamed of by physicians since Hippocrates. By understanding and manipulating this vast new cellular communications network we hold the keys to an acne- and disease-free future.

Appendix A
RECIPES FOR THE ACNE PRESCRIPTION

Most people assume that a diet regimen that is good for them must also necessarily taste blah, ordinary. That's not so with my program. My 28-Day Anti-Acne Diet is full of foods that are healthful and delicious.

I am especially fortunate that many of the recipes presented here were created exclusively for *The Acne Prescription* by award-winning executive chef Bernard Guillas. All the following recipes make liberal use of foods that are beneficial to people with acne. Chef Bernard presides over the Marine Room and the Shores Restaurant at the La Jolla Beach & Tennis Club in La Jolla, California. Prior to coming to the United States, Chef Bernard learned his craft in his native France and later honed his skills in such exotic locales as French Guyana—all of whose distinct regional influences imbue his cuisine with a unique and piquant flair.

Chef Bernard has provided recipes for breakfast, lunch, and dinner with a few desserts included as a special treat. Many of these recipes are to be made to the highest gourmet standards, while others are very simple and easy to prepare. All possess the understated elegance and sublime flavor that have made Chef Bernard renowned the world over.

You will notice that occasionally a recipe will call for a small amount of fruit juice. As my readers know, I do not advocate drinking juices as they can rapidly elevate the blood sugar and trigger an insulin response. (For more details on this please refer to Chapter One.) However, in these instances the amount of juice is small and used in combination with many other ingredients, thereby rendering it much less likely to cause any negative effects. One exception is PomWonderful pomegranate juice. This slightly tart, delicious juice is low in sugars and very high in antioxidants.

Whenever possible, try to use fresh, organic ingredients; this will ensure that you will enjoy the richest flavor and highest nutritional value.

A number of these ingredients may not be familiar or available to you. Many of them can be found in Oriental or gourmet markets. However, if you can't find a particular ingredient but want to make the recipe, I encourage you to substitute a readily available ingredient rather than forgo a chance to try a new and exciting recipe.

In the words of Chef Bernard: "A good cook is a sorcerer who dispenses happiness on a plate."

Chef Bernard and I both wish you bon appetit!

Breakfast, Brunch, and Lunch Dishes

Tropical Yogurt Strawberries, Pink Grapefruit, and Kiwi Frappé

2 large pink grapefruits, peeled and segmented
2 kiwis, peeled and diced
½ cup quartered strawberries
1 cup unflavored whole-milk yogurt
½ cup sparkling water
6 ice cubes
Juice and zest of 1 lemon
½ teaspoon freshly grated ginger

1. In a stainless steel mixing bowl combine grapefruit, kiwi, and strawberries.

2. Cover bowl with plastic wrap, and place in freezer for 30 minutes.

3. Remove bowl from freezer. Place fruit mixture in a blender or food processor. Add yogurt, sparkling water, ice cubes, lemon juice and zest, and ginger. Blend until smooth and frothy.

Presentation
4 strawberries
4 spears lemongrass
4 sprigs mint

1. Skewer each strawberry with 1 lemongrass spear.

2. Pour frappé into four tall, chilled glasses.

3. Garnish each serving with a lemongrass-strawberry skewer and a mint sprig.

YIELD: 4 SERVINGS

Almond-Flour Pancakes with Berry Compote and Cantaloupe Balls

Berry Compote

¼ cup diced strawberries

¼ cup raspberries

¼ cup blackberries

¼ cup blueberries

¼ cup boysenberries

Pinch star anise powder

Pinch cayenne pepper

1. In a mixing bowl combine the berries and the spices. Set aside. Let sit one hour at room temperature.

Almond-Flour Pancakes

⅔ cup whole-curd cottage cheese

3 large eggs

½ cup ground almond meal (or almond flour)

⅛ teaspoon vanilla extract

⅛ teaspoon ground cinnamon

2 tablespoons oat bran

1. In a large mixing bowl combine all ingredients: the cottage cheese, eggs, almond meal, vanilla, and cinnamon. Beat until smooth.

2. Heat a nonstick griddle or large nonstick skillet.

3. For each pancake, pour about 3 tablespoons of batter onto the griddle or skillet.

4. Sprinkle each pancake with oat bran.

5. Cook pancakes 1 to 2 minutes until puffed and dry around edges. Turn and cook other side until golden brown. Keep warm in oven.

Presentation
1 cantaloupe
6 sprigs mint

1. Cut cantaloupe in half. Remove seeds. Use a melon baller to scoop flesh from the cantaloupe.

2. For each serving, place three pancakes in the center of a plate. Spoon berry compote on top. Garnish with mint sprig. Surround pancakes with melon balls.

YIELD: **6** SERVINGS

Baja Jack Cheese Crabmeat Omelette with Tomato and Apple Salsa Fresca, and Avocado

Tomato and Apple Salsa Fresca
3 medium tomatoes, diced
1 small apple, peeled, cored, and diced
¼ cup scallions, chopped
1 small jalapeño pepper, seeded and finely chopped
2 tablespoons finely chopped cilantro
2 tablespoons fresh lime juice
½ teaspoon salt

1. In a glass bowl combine all ingredients. Cover.

2. Refrigerate at least 1 hour to blend flavors.

3. Spoon into four ramekins.

Crabmeat Omelette
½ pound fresh or canned crabmeat
¼ cup finely chopped red bell peppers

2 teaspoons chopped chives
Juice of 1 lemon
8 large eggs
4 tablespoons water
1 teaspoon extra virgin olive oil
8 slices jack cheese
Sea salt and freshly ground black pepper

1. Preheat the broiler.

2. Pick over the crabmeat. In a small bowl, combine crabmeat, bell peppers, chives, and lemon juice. Set aside.

3. In a small bowl, whip eggs and water until frothy.

4. In a small nonstick skillet heat the olive oil. Add half egg mixture. Stir briefly with fork. Allow eggs to begin to set at edges. Lift omelette edges and tilt the pan to allow the uncooked egg mixture to flow beneath the cooked layer. Cook 4–5 minutes until the eggs are almost set but still moist.

5. Spread half the crabmeat mixture over half the omelette. Season to taste with salt and pepper.

6. Fold the other half of the omelette over the crabmeat filling.

7. Top with 4 slices of jack cheese.

8. Place under the hot broiler for 30 seconds, or until the cheese melts.

9. Remove from broiler and invert onto warmed plate.

Presentation
1 avocado, quartered, and sliced into fans
4 sprigs cilantro

1. Divide each omelette in half. Place each half on a warmed plate.

2. Serve each omelette with a ramekin of tomato and apple salsa. Garnish the omelette with avocado fan and cilantro sprig.

YIELD: 4 SERVINGS

Chef Bernard's Granola with Yogurt, Strawberries, and Blackberries

Granola

1 cup rolled oats

⅓ cup oat bran

¼ cup coarsely chopped macadamia nuts

¼ cup coarsely chopped pecans

¼ cup sliced almonds

2 tablespoons shelled pumpkin seeds

Zest of 1 orange

⅓ cup grapeseed oil

2 teaspoons vanilla extract

1 teaspoon almond extract

½ teaspoon lemongrass powder

¼ teaspoon ground cardamom

¼ teaspoon ground ginger

¼ teaspoon star anise powder

¼ cup shredded unsweetened coconut

1. Preheat oven to 225°F.

2. In large mixing bowl combine rolled oats, oat bran, macadamia nuts, pecans, almonds, pumpkin seeds, and orange zest.

3. Add grapeseed oil, vanilla and almond extracts, and spices. Rub mixture between your palms to thoroughly coat the mixture with the oil and flavorings.

4. Spread the mixture thinly and evenly on two 10 x 15 baking sheets.

5. Bake 1½ hours, until golden, stirring occasionally.

6. Remove from oven. Let cool to room temperature. Toss with coconut on the baking sheet.

Presentation

3 cups unflavored whole milk yogurt

1 pint strawberries

6 nectarines

6 sprigs mint

1. Wash, dry, and quarter the strawberries. Cut the nectarines in half and remove the pits. Cut nectarines into thin wedges.

2. Divide yogurt among six chilled bowls. Top with portion of granola. Garnish with the fruit and a mint sprig.

YIELD: **6** SERVINGS

Eggs Benedict with Smoked Salmon, Seared Tomatoes, Asparagus, and Meyer Lemon–Olive Oil Hollandaise

Poached Eggs
2 tablespoons white wine vinegar
12 large eggs

1. Bring 2 quarts of water to a boil in large shallow pan.

2. Add the white wine vinegar to the water. Lower the heat to a simmer.

3. Break 6 of the eggs into six small bowls.

4. Gently slide each egg into the simmering water.

5. Poach until the whites are firm, about 2 minutes.

6. With a slotted spoon remove the eggs from the water. Drain on a paper towel.

7. Repeat with the remaining six eggs.

8. Keep warm in oven.

Meyer Lemon–Olive Oil Hollandaise
4 egg yolks
2 tablespoons water
Juice and zest of 1 Meyer lemon
⅓ cup extra virgin olive oil
Sea salt and freshly ground black pepper

1. In a stainless steel bowl combine egg yolks, water, and lemon zest and juice.

2. In a double boiler set over simmering water. Whisk yolk mixture until light and fluffy. Remove top of double boiler from heat.

3. Slowly add and whisk olive oil into the yolk mixture. Season to taste with salt and pepper.

Seared Tomatoes
4 medium tomatoes
1 tablespoon extra virgin olive oil
¼ teaspoon paprika
Sea salt and freshly ground black pepper

1. Cut each tomato into 3 slices.

2. Brush cut sides with olive oil.

3. Season to taste with paprika, salt, and pepper.

4. Place large nonstick skillet over high heat.

5. Sear tomato slices, about 1 minute per side.

Presentation
12 slices smoked salmon
24 asparagus spears
3 tablespoons finely minced chives

1. Trim and peel asparagus. Steam spears 4 to 5 minutes.

2. For each serving place two tomatoes on warmed plate. Top each tomato with a slice of smoked salmon. Top each salmon slice with 1 poached egg. Spoon hollandaise over each egg. Garnish with 4 asparagus spears and a sprinkling of minced chives.

Yield: **6 servings**

Scrambled Eggs with Parmesan and
Warm Mushroom Salad

8 large eggs
3 tablespoons milk
1 tablespoon chopped chervil
Sea salt and freshly ground white pepper
1 tablespoon extra virgin olive oil
¼ cup grated Parmesan

1. In a large mixing bowl whisk together eggs, milk, and chervil. Season to taste with salt and pepper.

2. In medium skillet heat olive oil over medium heat. Pour in egg mixture.

3. Let sit 30 seconds, then stir occasionally until large curds form.

4. When eggs are firm but still fairly moist, add the cheese. Stir gently to blend.

Warm Mushroom Salad
1 tablespoon extra virgin olive oil
⅓ cup pearl onions, peeled
¼ cup turkey bacon, diced
¼ cup quartered cremini mushrooms
¼ cup quartered oyster mushrooms
¼ cup quartered white button mushrooms
¼ cup vegetable stock
¼ cup scallions, thinly sliced on the diagonal
1 tablespoon chopped fresh parsley
1 teaspoon chopped fresh thyme
1 large tomato, diced
Sea salt and freshly ground black pepper

1. In large skillet heat the olive oil over medium heat.

2. Add pearl onions and turkey bacon. Cook until bacon is rendered and onions are golden.

3. Add all the mushrooms. Cook 30 seconds.

4. Add vegetable stock, scallions, parsley, and thyme.

5. Remove from heat. Add diced tomato. Toss.

6. Season to taste with salt and pepper. Set aside.

Presentation
4 sprigs chervil
2 tablespoons hazelnut oil

1. For each serving spoon scrambled eggs into a mound in center of warmed pasta bowl. Surround with warm mushroom salad. Garnish with chervil. Drizzle with hazelnut oil.

YIELD: 4 SERVINGS

Entrées with Accompaniments

Spiced Diver Scallops with Ecuadorian Tabouleh and Lemon Myrtle Oil

Spiced Scallops
¼ cup toasted almonds
½ teaspoon sea salt
¼ teaspoon lemongrass powder
⅛ teaspoon togarashi pepper mix *
10 fennel seeds
18 scallops, U-10 size, extralarge
2 tablespoons chopped fresh parsley
2 tablespoons extra virgin olive oil

1. In a spice grinder, pulverize almonds, salt, lemongrass powder, togarashi pepper mix, and fennel seeds.

---

*A seven-spice mixture that includes red chiles, sesame seeds, seaweed flakes, poppy seeds, and orange peel. Available in Oriental and gourmet food markets.

2. In a large bowl, toss scallops with spice mix and parsley.

3. Heat the olive oil in large nonstick skillet over high heat. Add half the scallops. Cook 1 minute. Turn. Cook additional 1 minute, or until done. Remove scallops from pan and set aside. Cook the remaining scallops.

Ecuadorian Tabouleh

2 cups quinoa*

4 cups water

¼ cup chopped red onion

½ cup chopped cilantro

½ cup chopped fresh mint

½ cup chopped fresh parsley

⅓ cup extra virgin olive oil

2 tablespoons lemon juice

3 tablespoons fresh lime juice

1 avocado, peeled, pitted, and diced

4 tomatoes, peeled, seeded, and diced

2 pepino melons, peeled, seeded, and diced

Sea salt and freshly ground black pepper

1. Wash the quinoa under running water. Place in medium pan. Add the water and bring to boil. Reduce heat to low. Cover and simmer until liquid is absorbed, approximately 10 to 15 minutes.

2. Remove from heat; quinoa will be somewhat translucent. Fluff with fork, and transfer quinoa to large bowl. Let cool to room temperature.

3. In a mixing bowl combine red onion, cilantro, mint, parsley, olive oil, and lemon and lime juices.

4. Add avocado, tomatoes, and melon.

5. Add mixture to quinoa. Toss gently. Season to taste with salt and pepper.

★ Quinoa is an ancient grain that contains more protein than any other grain: an average of 16.2 percent, compared with 7.5 percent for rice, 9.9 percent for millet, and 14 percent for wheat. Some varieties of quinoa are more than 20 percent protein. The protein in quinoa is of an unusually high quality. It is a complete protein, with an essential amino acid balance close to the ideal. Courtesy of Quinoa Corporation, www.quinoa.net.

Lemon Myrtle Oil

½ cup extra virgin olive oil

20 basil leaves

5 drops lemon myrtle oil

Sea salt and freshly ground black pepper

1. In heavy skillet heat the olive oil. When oil is hot, fry basil leaves crisp. Do not overfry or you will burn the chlorophyll and lose bright-green color.

2. Set aside the pan and let the basil and oil cool to room temperature. Place oil and basil in blender. Season with salt and pepper to taste. Blend well at high speed. Add the lemon myrtle oil.

Presentation

½ cup small-leaved arugula

6 sprigs fresh parsley

1. For each serving, pack tabouleh into a 2-ounce timbale. Unmold in the center of warmed plate.

2. Place three scallops, evenly spaced, around tabouleh. Drizzle with lemon myrtle oil. Top the tabouleh with small mound of arugula.

3. Garnish with parsley.

YIELD: **6** SERVINGS

Smoked Salmon Rillette with Butter Lettuce, Radish, and Hearts of Palm Salad, and Blood Orange Vinaigrette

Smoked Salmon Rillette

4 ounces fresh salmon fillet, boned and skinned

4 ounces smoked salmon

1 teaspoon fresh lime or lemon juice

½ cup unflavored whole milk yogurt

2 tablespoons finely chopped chives

½ teaspoon chopped mint

Sea salt and freshly ground black pepper

1. Steam fresh salmon, approximately 8 minutes. Place on paper towel. Set aside. Let cool.

2. Coarsely chop smoked salmon. Place in mixing bowl. Combine with lemon or lime juice, yogurt, and chives.

3. Flake steamed salmon. Fold into smoked salmon mixture. Divide into six ramekins. Chill two hours.

Butter Lettuce Salad

1 head butter lettuce
1 small bunch radishes, thinly sliced
6 medium hearts of palm, cut into slices on the diagonal
Juice and zest of 1 blood orange
1 teaspoon white wine vinegar
¼ teaspoon sea salt
3 tablespoons hazelnut oil

1. Toss together lettuce, radishes, and hearts of palm.

2. In a mixing bowl combine orange juice and zest, vinegar, and salt. Whisk in hazelnut oil.

3. Pour over salad. Toss.

Presentation

¼ cup toasted almonds
2 blood oranges, peeled, separated into segments

1. Divide salad among six chilled plates.

2. Unmold a ramekin of salmon rillette in the center of each salad.

3. Garnish with toasted almonds and orange segments.

YIELD: **6** SERVINGS

Steamed Black Mussels with Turkey Bacon, Japanese Eggplant, and Shiitake Mushrooms

1 tablespoon extra virgin olive oil

½ cup diced turkey bacon

1 Japanese eggplant, diced

¼ cup chopped shallots

6 pounds black mussels, cleaned, beards removed

½ cup sauvignon blanc

1 cup shiitake mushrooms, stems removed, quartered

¼ teaspoon turmeric

¼ teaspoon star anise powder

1 teaspoon chopped fresh oregano

Zest of 1 lemon

Freshly ground black pepper

3 tablespoons heavy cream

¼ cup minced chervil

1. In large stockpot heat the olive oil over medium heat. Add turkey bacon, eggplant, and shallots. Cook until eggplant is tender.

2. Add mussels, sauvignon blanc, mushrooms, turmeric, star anise, oregano, lemon zest, and black pepper. Cover. Cook over medium-high heat 3 minutes, until liquid starts to simmer.

3. Uncover. Add cream. With a slotted spoon toss mussel shells so they cook evenly. Cover. Cook until shells open, about 5 minutes.

4. Using a slotted spoon, remove mussels and place in warmed deep, serving platter. Pour broth over mussels. Sprinkle with chervil.

YIELD: **6 SERVINGS**

Pomegranate Citrus–Glazed Apricot- and Garlic-Roasted Chicken with Apple-Spinach Stuffing and Garden Vegetables

Pomegranate-Citrus Glaze
Juice of 3 pomegranates
Juice of 3 mandarin oranges
2 tablespoons sherry vinegar
1 teaspoon lavender flowers

1. In a small saucepan combine all glaze ingredients.

2. Over medium heat bring to boil, then lower heat.

3. Simmer until liquid is syrupy and reduce by two thirds. Set aside.

Apricot- and Garlic-Roasted Chicken
1 head garlic
3 tablespoons extra virgin olive oil
½ cup finely chopped apricots
2 tablespoons finely chopped lemon thyme
1 tablespoon finely chopped sage
4½ to 5 pound free-range chicken
Sea salt and freshly ground black pepper
2 Granny Smith apples, peeled, cored, and quartered
2 cups white button mushrooms
2 cups packed fresh spinach leaves
½ cup sun-dried sour cherries

1. Preheat oven to 375°F.

2. Cut ½ inch off the top of the garlic head. Place on large sheet of heavy-duty aluminum foil. Drizzle with 1 tablespoon of the olive oil. Seal foil tightly around garlic. Roast until cloves are tender, 30 to 35 minutes.

3. When garlic is cool enough to handle, squeeze the pulp out of each clove into a mixing bowl. Mash with the apricots, lemon thyme, and sage.

4. Gently separate and loosen the chicken skin over the breasts and legs. With your fingers, spread garlic mixture between the chicken skin and breast and leg meat.

5. Rub 1 tablespoon of the olive oil evenly over the chicken. Season chicken, inside and out, with salt and pepper.

6. In large bowl combine apples, mushrooms, spinach, and cherries. Stuff into chicken cavity.

7. Put chicken in roasting pan, breast side up. Place pan in the center of the oven.

Garden Vegetables

1 cup cipollini onions, peeled
18 small brussels sprouts
18 baby turnips, peeled
12 baby bok choy
6 canned artichoke hearts, quartered
3 tablespoons extra virgin olive oil

1. In a large bowl toss the vegetables with olive oil.

2. After the chicken has cooked 30 minutes, remove its pan from oven, surround chicken with the vegetables, and return pan to oven.

3. Continue roasting for about 1¼ hours, basting with pomegranate-citrus glaze every 10 minutes. Turn the vegetables periodically to ensure even cooking. Roast chicken until juices run clear at the thickest part of the thigh.

Presentation

¼ cup white wine
½ cup chicken stock
Sea salt and freshly ground black pepper

1. Remove chicken from roasting pan and place on serving platter. Scatter the vegetables over the chicken.

2. Place the roasting pan on the stove top over medium-high heat. Stir in white wine and chicken stock, and reduce liquid by one third. Season to taste with salt and pepper.

3. Strain. Transfer to sauce boat and serve with chicken.

YIELD: **6** SERVINGS

Tofu Vegetable Stir-fry with Yuzu Sauce

Tofu

1 15–16 oz. package firm tofu

2 tablespoons mirin (Japanese rice wine)

2 tablespoons julienned pickled ginger

2 tablespoons water

2 tablespoons low-sodium soy sauce

1 tablespoon rice vinegar

1 clove garlic, crushed

1. Gently rinse tofu under running water. Pat dry.

2. Slice into 6 portions and place in large bowl.

3. In a mixing bowl combine the mirin, ginger, water, soy sauce, rice vinegar, and garlic. Pour over tofu slices. Let stand 2 hours.

4. Drain, reserving the liquid.

5. Cut tofu into cubes and set aside.

Yuzu Sauce

1 tablespoon chopped cilantro

1 tablespoon yuzu* juice

Zest of 1 orange

Hot chili oil (to taste)

1. Add the cilantro, yuzu juice, orange zest, and chili oil to the reserved marinade.

2. Set aside.

---

* Yuzu is a citrus fruit common in Japanese kitchens. The flavor of the juice is similar to grapefruit but has overtones of mandarin orange.

Vegetable stir-fry
⅔ cup honshimeji mushrooms
½ cup cauliflower florets
½ cup broccoli florets
½ cup sliced bamboo shoots
½ cup snow peas, cut in half on the diagonal
½ cup bean sprouts
½ cup julienned red bell pepper
1 teaspoon grated orange peel
½ teaspoon sesame seeds
½ teaspoon mustard seeds
Sea salt and freshly ground black pepper
2 tablespoons extra virgin olive oil

1. In a large bowl combine the vegetables, orange peel, and sesame and mustard seeds. Season to taste with salt and pepper.

2. Heat the oil in frying pan or wok. Sauté the vegetables 5 to 8 minutes over high heat until tender-crisp, stirring constantly. Add the marinated tofu. Toss gently with the vegetables. Add yuzu sauce. Cover. Heat through.

Presentation
3 tablespoons pine nuts
6 sprigs cilantro

1. Divide tofu and vegetables among 6 shallow serving bowls.

2. Garnish with pine nuts and cilantro sprigs.

How to toast pine nuts: Preheat oven to 350°F. Place pine nuts in a shallow glass baking dish. Stir occasionally. When nuts turn a warm golden brown they are ready—approximate time is 10 minutes.

YIELD: **6** SERVINGS

Turkey Sausage–Filled Portobello Mushrooms with Red Grape–Apple Chutney and Spoon Spinach Salad

Portobello Mushrooms

6 portobello mushrooms (approximately 5 inches in
    diameter)
¼ cup balsamic vinegar
¼ cup extra virgin olive oil
1 tablespoon finely chopped fresh rosemary
Sea salt and freshly ground black pepper

1. Preheat oven to 375°F.

2. Clean mushrooms thoroughly with damp towel or soft brush. Remove stems. With a spoon remove black gills from underside of cap.

3. In a mixing bowl, combine vinegar, olive oil, rosemary, and salt and pepper. Whisk.

4. Add mushroom caps and marinate for 15 minutes.

5. Remove mushrooms from marinade. Place on a baking sheet, stem side up. Bake for 10 minutes. Remove from oven. Let cool.

Red Grape–Apple Chutney

1 tablespoon extra virgin olive oil
¼ cup minced leeks, white parts only
1 green apple, peeled, cored, and finely diced
1 tablespoon yellow mustard seeds
Juice of 2 lemons
3 tablespoons unsweetened applesauce
¼ teaspoon cumin
Pinch cayenne pepper
⅓ cup quartered seedless red grapes
¼ cup pine nuts, toasted
Sea salt and freshly ground black pepper

1. In a large skillet heat olive oil over medium heat. Add leeks, apple, and mustard seeds. Cook without browning, 2 minutes.

2. Add lemon juice, applesauce, cumin, and cayenne pepper. Simmer over low heat for 15 minutes, until mixture has thickened. Fold in grapes and toasted pine nuts. Set aside. Cool.

Preparation

1. OVEN Wash and dry the peppers. Cut off the tops, and cut in half, removing seeds and membranes. Place on a baking sheet in the oven and put under the broiler until the skin is blackened and blistered. Place them in a heavy-duty sealable plastic bag with the seal tightly closed for 20 minutes. Do not skip this step as this "steaming" period is what makes the skin easily removed from the peppers. Peel the peppers and remove the skin (it should slip right off at this point), and cut the peppers into the size of strips you desire.

2. GRILL On a charcoal barbecue or a gas-fired barbecue place the whole peppers on the grill and roast [turning occasionally] until the skins are blackened. Remove from the grill and let cool until they can be handled for peeling off the blackened skin. Clean out the seeds and veins and use whole or cut into needed size.

Turkey Sausage Stuffing

6 medium turkey sausages, removed from casings,
    meat crumbled
¼ cup grated Parmesan
2 tablespoons finely chopped fresh parsley
3 tablespoons chopped roasted red bell peppers
1 tablespoon finely chopped fresh oregano
1 teaspoon finely chopped fresh thyme
Sea salt and freshly ground black pepper

1. Preheat broiler.

2. In a mixing bowl combine all ingredients. Season to taste with salt and pepper.

3. Divide mixture into 6 portions. Spoon into mushroom caps.

4. Bake under broiler, 3 to 4 minutes, or until golden brown.

Spoon Spinach Salad

1 cup spoon spinach, washed and patted dry

1 cup frisée

2 large Belgian endives, washed, patted dry, leaves cut on
    diagonal

3 tablespoons pistachio oil

2 tablespoons rice wine vinegar

Sea salt and freshly ground black pepper

1. Combine greens in large mixing bowl.

2. In a small bowl, whisk together pistachio oil and rice wine vinegar.
Season to taste with salt and pepper.

3. Pour dressing over salad and toss.

Presentation

1. For each serving, place a mound of salad in the center of a plate.
Lean 1 stuffed mushroom against the salad. Top the mushroom with 1 tablespoon of grape-apple chutney.

YIELD: **6** SERVINGS

Wild King Salmon and Tuna Sashimi with Exotic Fruit Relish

Exotic Fruit Relish

2 Asian pears, peeled, cored, and finely diced

6 lychee nuts, shelled, pitted, and diced

3 red plums, pitted and diced

1 kiwi, peeled and diced

¼ cup tangerine juice

1 teaspoon chopped cilantro

1 teaspoon grated fresh ginger

Pinch togarashi pepper mix

1. In a large bowl combine all ingredients.

2. Set aside for 30 minutes.

Wild King Salmon and Tuna Sashimi
8-ounce fillet wild king salmon, sashimi quality, skin off, pin
bone removed
8 ounces ahi tuna, sashimi quality, skin off, blood line
removed

1. Place salmon fillet on cutting board. Thinly slice on the diagonal into six portions.

2. Place a sliced salmon fillet between two large sheets of plastic wrap. With a wooden mallet gently pound until thin and flat. Repeat with remaining salmon fillets.

3. Slice ahi tuna into ⅛-inch-thick slices.

4. Refrigerate salmon and tuna.

Presentation
Juice of 3 limes
2 tablespoons pumpkin seed oil
Sea salt and freshly ground black pepper
2 tablespoons freshly grated Parmesan
2 tablespoons finely chopped chives
6 chive blossoms
18 basil leaves

1. Remove salmon and tuna from refrigerator.

2. For each salmon fillet, carefully peel plastic wrap from one side. Place fish side down on a chilled serving plate. Gently peel off remaining plastic wrap.

3. Mound 2 tablespoons fruit relish in center of each salmon portion. Arrange sliced ahi tuna around the relish.

4. Drizzle everything with lime juice and pumpkin seed oil. Season to taste with salt and pepper.

5. Sprinkle with Parmesan and chives.

6. Garnish with a chive blossom and 3 basil leaves.

YIELD: **6** SERVINGS

Barbecued Jumbo Baja Prawns with Grilled Belgian Endive and Mandarin–Avocado Relish

Prawns
2 pounds jumbo prawns, preferably Mexican, U-10 size
⅓ cup pink grapefruit juice
1 teaspoon fresh thyme, finely chopped
½ teaspoon cumin
½ teaspoon green curry
1 teaspoon fresh mint, finely chopped
¼ cup walnut oil
Sea salt and freshly ground black pepper

1. Butterfly prawns, and set aside.

2. Make the marinade. In small bowl, combine grapefruit juice, thyme, cumin, curry, mint, and walnut oil. Season to taste with salt and pepper.

3. Place shrimp in square baking dish and add the marinade. Let stand 15 minutes.

4. Pour off marinade, strain, and reserve.

Belgian Endive
½ cup extra virgin olive oil
Juice and zest of 1 blood orange
2 tablespoons brown rice vinegar
1 teaspoon chopped fresh lemon thyme
Pinch cayenne pepper
Sea salt
6 small Belgian endives, halved

1. Preheat a barbecue.

2. Make a marinade. Combine olive oil, orange juice and zest, rice vinegar, lemon thyme, cayenne pepper, and salt in mixing bowl.

3. Add endives and marinate 20 minutes.

4. Place endives on hot grill, cut sides down. Grill 5 minutes. Turn over. Grill additional 5 minutes. Cook until tender, basting frequently with marinade.

Mandarin–Avocado Relish

2 avocados, peeled, pitted, and diced
1 mandarin orange, peeled and segmented
½ cup jicama,* julienned
1 teaspoon cilantro leaves, finely chopped
Juice of 1 lemon
Sea salt and freshly ground black pepper
Dash Tabasco

1. In a large nonmetal bowl combine avocado, mandarin orange, jicama, and cilantro. Mix with a wooden spatula.

2. Add lemon juice; season to taste with salt, pepper, and Tabasco.

3. Set aside.

Presentation

Mint sprigs
Thyme sprigs

1. Place shrimp on grill or barbecue cut side down. Cook over hot coals two minutes. Turn shrimp. Cook until opaque, being careful to not overcook.

2. For each serving, place 2 endive halves, overlapping, in the center of each plate. Spoon avocado–mango relish in center of endive.

3. Arrange 3 grilled shrimp around the relish, atop endive.

4. Whisk reserved marinade vigorously. Drizzle over shrimp.

5. Garnish with several mint and thyme sprigs.

YIELD: 6 SERVINGS (AS AN APPETIZER)

---

* Jicama is a white-fleshed tuber, shaped like a turnip, that can weigh from half a pound to five pounds or more. It has a thin brown skin and crisp, juicy flesh similar in texture to an apple's. Although jicama can be used in some of the same ways as a potato, it is less starchy and lower in calories (a cup of sliced jicama has about 50 calories, 11 grams of carbohydrate, and 5.9 grams of fiber). The vegetable is a good source of vitamin C and also contains some potassium, iron, and calcium.

Summer Gazpacho with Jumbo Bay Shrimp and Crabmeat Salad

Gazpacho
3 cups diced heirloom tomatoes
2 tablespoons chopped cilantro
¼ cup chopped red onion
2 tablespoons extra virgin olive oil
1 cup chicken stock, chilled
1 clove garlic, minced
1 tablespoon rice vinegar
1 teaspoon sambal (Asian chile sauce)
Juice of 1 Meyer lemon
1 cup peeled, seeded, and finely diced cucumber
½ cup peeled, cored, and finely diced apple
¼ cup minced scallions
Sea salt and freshly ground black pepper

1. Place tomatoes, cilantro, onion, olive oil, chicken stock, garlic, rice vinegar, sambal, and lemon juice in a blender. Pulse at high speed approximately 15 seconds, until coarsely chopped.

2. Transfer to glass mixing bowl. Stir in cucumber, apples, and scallions. Season to taste with salt and pepper. Refrigerate approximately 1 hour.

Shrimp and Crabmeat Salad
⅔ cup crabmeat, cooked
½ cup jumbo bay shrimps, cooked
3 tablespoons verjus*
2 tablespoons hazelnut oil
Sea salt and freshly ground black pepper

* Verjus is the tart, unfermented juice of unripe wine grapes. It is used to add acidity to foods, but unlike vinegar and lemon juice, it happens to be very compatible with wine, as it is a grape product.

1. In a mixing bowl toss crabmeat and shrimp with verjus and hazelnut oil.

2. Season to taste with salt and pepper.

Presentation
6 sprigs opal basil
12 yellow teardrop tomatoes, halved
12 red teardrop tomatoes, halved

1. For each serving, pour gazpacho into a chilled soup bowl or large pasta plate. Spoon a portion of shellfish salad into center of each bowl.

2. Garnish with opal basil and teardrop tomato halves. Serve chilled.

YIELD: **6 SERVINGS**

East-West Chicken Breast and Green-Curry Barley Casserole with Green Beans

East-West Chicken Breast
Juice and zest of 3 large oranges
¾ cup chopped shallots
¼ cup low-sodium soy sauce
3 tablespoons extra virgin olive oil
1½ tablespoons chopped fresh mint
1 tablespoon sesame oil
1½ teaspoons grated fresh ginger
½ teaspoon tamarind powder
1 stalk lemongrass heart, finely chopped
Sea salt and freshly ground black pepper
6 8-ounce boneless, skinless chicken breasts

1. Make a marinade. In a large bowl combine juice and zest of oranges, shallots, soy sauce, olive oil, mint, sesame oil, ginger tamarind powder, and lemongrass. Season to taste with salt and pepper.

2. Add chicken breasts.

3. Marinate approximately 1½ hours. Set aside.

Green-Curry Barley Casserole with Green Beans

1½ tablespoons extra virgin olive oil

½ cup finely diced yellow onions

⅓ cup quartered white button mushrooms

1 teaspoon chopped fresh thyme

1 teaspoon green curry paste

1 cup pearl barley

3 cups vegetable stock

1 cup green beans, steamed, cut diagonally into ½-inch pieces

¼ cup toasted cashews

Sea salt and freshly ground black pepper

1. Preheat oven to 350°F.

2. Heat olive oil in large ovenproof skillet. Add onions and mushrooms. Cook without browning, about two minutes.

3. Add thyme and curry paste. Cook 1 minute.

4. Add barley and vegetable stock. Bring to boil.

5. Cover skillet. Place in preheated oven. Cook 45 minutes, until liquid is absorbed.

6. Remove skillet from oven. Fold in green beans and cashews. Season to taste with salt and pepper.

Preparation

Remove chicken breasts from marinade, reserving marinade. Cut each breast into 2 lobes. Brush a large skillet or grill generously with olive oil. Cook chicken breasts over moderate heat for approximately 5 minutes on each side, or until done.

Sauce

Reserved marinade

1 tablespoon walnut oil

Sea salt and freshly ground black pepper

1. Pour 1½ cups of the reserved marinade mixture in medium saucepan over moderate heat. Cook until liquid is reduced by half.

2. Strain through fine sieve into a bowl. Whisk in walnut oil. Season to taste.

Presentation

3 oranges, peeled and cut into 10 segments

18 stalks asparagus, peeled and steamed

6 sprigs fresh mint

1. For each serving, place barley mixture on a plate.

2. Top with 2 chicken breast lobes.

3. Arrange 5 orange segments around the chicken. Ladle sauce over chicken and barley.

4. Garnish with steamed asparagus and a mint sprig.

Yield: **6 servings**

Fennel Pollen–Spiced Chicken Paillard with Heirloom Vegetable Ratatouille and Red Lentils

Fennel Pollen—Spiced Chicken Paillard

6 6-ounce boneless, skinless chicken breasts

¼ cup extra virgin olive oil

¼ cup chopped flat leaf parsley

Zest of 2 lemons

1 teaspoon fennel pollen*

⅛ teaspoon ground cumin

Sea salt and freshly ground black pepper

1. Place each chicken breast between two pieces of heavy-duty plastic wrap.

2. Pound each chicken breast with a meat mallet until it is about ¼ inch thick.

3. Remove zest from the lemons, reserving the lemons.

4. Make the marinade. In a large shallow dish, combine olive oil, pars-

---

* Fennel pollen is harvested from wild fennel plants in California. It possesses an aroma similar to anise, and complements beef, pork, poultry, seafood, or vegetables.

ley, lemon zest, fennel pollen, and cumin. Season to taste with salt and pepper. Place chicken paillards in marinade. Turn to coat.

5. Heat large nonstick skillet over medium heat. Remove chicken from marinade. Sear chicken paillards 3 minutes per side, or until golden brown.

Heirloom Vegetable Ratatouille
4 tablespoons extra virgin olive oil
½ cup peeled, diced eggplant
½ cup diced onion
½ cup zucchini
4 medium heirloom tomatoes, diced
2 tablespoons minced garlic
1 red bell pepper, roasted, seeded, and julienned
   (see page 190)
1 yellow bell pepper, roasted, seeded, and julienned
1 orange bell pepper, roasted, seeded, and julienned
1 tablespoon chopped basil
4 sprigs opal basil
Sea salt and freshly ground black pepper

1. Heat 2 tablespoons of the olive oil in large skillet until very hot.

2. Add eggplant and sauté over medium heat, stirring constantly.

3. Add remaining olive oil, onion, and zucchini. Cook 2 minutes.

4. Add tomatoes and garlic. Cook 10 minutes, or until liquid has evaporated.

5. Add julienned peppers and basils. Season to taste with salt and pepper. Set aside.

Red Lentils
2½ cups vegetable stock
1 cup red lentils
2 tablespoons chopped chives
1 tablespoon almond oil
Juice of 2 lemons

Dash Tabasco

Sea salt and freshly ground black pepper

1. In large pot bring vegetable stock to boil.

2. Add lentils, and cook approximately 10 minutes.

3. Rinse lentils under cold water. Drain.

4. Stir in chives, almond oil, lemon juice, and Tabasco. Season to taste with salt and pepper.

5. Spoon lentil mixture into six ramekins.

Presentation

6 sprigs basil

2 tablespoons extra virgin olive oil

1. For each serving, place a portion of ratatouille on a warmed plate. Top with one chicken paillard.

2. Unmold a ramekin of red lentils and arrange beside chicken.

3. Garnish with basil sprigs. Drizzle with extra virgin olive oil.

YIELD: **6** SERVINGS

Feta and Spinach-Stuffed Chicken Breast with Warm Green Bean and Pear Salad and Grilled Heirloom Tomatoes

Feta and Spinach Stuffing

3 cups packed spoon spinach

2 tablespoons olive oil, not extra virgin

½ cup oyster mushrooms, thinly sliced

1 teaspoon chopped shallots

¾ cup feta

2 tablespoons chopped basil

Sea salt and freshly ground black pepper

1. Wash spinach and pat dry.

2. Heat olive oil in skillet over medium heat. Add mushrooms and shallots. Sauté for 2 minutes without browning.

3. Add spinach. Cook 1 minute, until wilted.

4. Remove from pan. Set aside. Let cool.

5. Combine spinach mixture with feta and basil. Season to taste with salt and pepper.

Chicken Breast

6 8-ounce boneless double chicken breasts
Sea salt and freshly ground black pepper
1 tablespoon olive oil
1 tablespoon chopped fresh oregano

1. Preheat oven to 375°F.

2. Season chicken to taste with salt and pepper.

3. Spread out chicken breasts flat on a cutting board and pound gently with a wooden mallet.

4. Divide feta-spinach stuffing into 6 portions and place one portion in center of each chicken breast. Roll breast tightly around stuffing.

5. Place chicken rolls, seam side down, in a cold skillet, and drizzle with olive oil. Season to taste with oregano, salt, and pepper.

6. Bake in oven 12 to 15 minutes, until juices run clear.

Warm Green Bean and Pear Salad

1½ tablespoons seasoned rice vinegar
⅓ cup lemon olive oil
Sea salt and freshly ground black pepper
1 pound green beans
1 pear, julienned
1 teaspoon chopped fresh tarragon

1. Make the vinaigrette. In a bowl whisk vinegar and oil until emulsified. Season to taste with salt and pepper.

2. Bring water to a boil in a skillet. Add salt. Add beans and cook until crisp-tender, approximately 5 to 8 minutes.

3. Drain beans, rinse in cold water, and drain again.

4. Transfer beans to a bowl and toss with pears, tarragon, and the vinaigrette until evenly coated.

Grilled Heirloom Tomatoes
3 large heirloom tomatoes
2 cloves garlic, minced
2 tablespoons finely chopped parsley
¼ cup extra virgin olive oil
2 tablespoons balsamic vinegar
Sea salt and freshly ground black pepper

1. Core tomatoes and cut in half horizontally. Place in baking dish, cut side up.

2. Make the marinade. In mixing bowl, combine garlic, parsley, olive oil, vinegar, salt, and pepper.

3. Pour marinade over tomatoes and let stand 15 minutes.

4. Remove tomatoes from dish. Reserve marinade. On hot grill, place tomatoes cut side down. Grill 2 to 3 minutes, or until lightly caramelized. Turn. Repeat.

5. Return grilled tomatoes to baking dish. Baste with reserved marinade.

6. Return to grill and cook for another 5 minutes.

Presentation

1. For each serving, mound green bean salad in center of warmed plate. Top with grilled tomato slice.

2. Cut each chicken breast into three pieces. Arrange around green bean salad.

3. Drizzle with reserved tomato marinade.

YIELD: **6** SERVINGS

Hawaiian Ahi Tuna Tartare on Daikon Radish Rounds with Quail Eggs and Tobiko Caviar

1 pound ahi tuna, sashimi grade #1, skin off, blood line
 removed
⅓ cup finely chopped shallots

4 tablespoons extra virgin olive oil

Juice of 2 Meyer lemons

Dash Tabasco

1 tablespoon chopped parsley

1 teaspoon capers

2 roma tomatoes, diced

1 tablespoon finely chopped Thai basil

Sea salt and freshly ground black pepper

1 medium daikon radish, peeled and cut into
   ⅛-inch-thick slices

12 quail eggs, hard-boiled, peeled, and halved
   (if you are unable to find quail eggs, substitute small
   chicken eggs)

2 tablespoons red tobiko caviar

6 sprigs chives, cut diagonally in 1-inch-long pieces

1. Finely chop ahi tuna and place in a chilled container.

2. In a small bowl whisk together shallots, olive oil, lemon juice, and Tabasco.

3. Add shallot mixture to ahi. Fold in parsley, capers, tomatoes, and chopped basil. Season to taste with salt and pepper.

4. Arrange daikon radish rounds on a large serving platter. Top each round with a dollop of ahi tuna mixture. Garnish each with half a hard-boiled quail egg topped with tobiko caviar and chives.

   YIELD: **6** SERVINGS

Leek and Chervil–Crusted Alaskan Halibut over Wilted Greens with Lemon-Scented Piperade

Leek and Chervil Crust

⅓ cup minced leeks, white part only

Sea salt and freshly ground black pepper

⅓ cup chopped chervil, washed and patted dry

2 tablespoons extra virgin olive oil

1. Wash and pat dry leeks. In skillet over medium heat cook leeks in olive oil until wilted. Season to taste with salt and pepper.

2. Place leeks in a mixing bowl; stir in chervil. Let cool.

Alaskan Halibut

6 7-ounce Alaskan halibut fillets
2 tablespoons extra virgin olive oil
Sea salt and freshly ground black pepper

1. Spread leek and chervil mixture on top of halibut fillets.

2. Heat olive oil in nonstick skillet at medium heat.

3. Place halibut, mixture side down, in skillet. Cook 3 minutes without browning.

4. Turn. Cook additional 3 minutes, or until done.

Wilted Greens

2 tablespoons extra virgin olive oil
1 teaspoon chopped shallots
2 cups packed arugula
2 cups packed spoon spinach
3 large red chard leaves, stems removed, chopped
¼ cup chopped basil
Sea salt and freshly ground black pepper

1. Heat olive oil in large skillet. Add shallots and cook without browning, about 2 minutes.

2. Add arugula, spinach, chard, and basil. Season to taste with salt and pepper. Cook 2 minutes until greens are wilted.

3. Drain in a colander.

Lemon-Scented Piperade

2 tablespoons plus ⅓ cup extra virgin olive oil
2 cloves garlic, cut into slivers
½ cup coarsely chopped onion
1 cup seeded, diced sweet bell pepper
1 cup peeled, seeded, diced tomato

1 peeled, seeded, diced lemon

Sea salt and freshly ground white pepper

20 pitted, chopped black niçoise olives

1. In medium saucepan over medium heat, heat 2 tablespoons of the olive oil. Add garlic, onions, and bell pepper. Cook 5 minutes. Do not allow vegetables to brown.

2. Add tomatoes and season with salt and pepper to taste. Bring to boil.

3. Lower heat. Cook 20 minutes, stirring occasionally.

4. Fold in lemon and niçoise olives. Cook 1 minute.

5. Remove from heat. Let stand 10 minutes. Pour in ⅓ cup of the extra virgin olive oil. Stir gently with wooden spoon. Season to taste.

Presentation

6 sprigs thyme

1. For each serving place wilted greens in center of warmed plate. Top with halibut fillet. Spoon piperade sauce around fillet.

2. Garnish with thyme sprig.

YIELD: **6 SERVINGS**

Lobster Spring Roll with Tangerine Soy Dipping Sauce

Lobster Spring Roll

¼ cup seasoned rice vinegar

½ teaspoon togarashi peppermix

Sea salt and freshly ground black pepper

1 cup julienned cucumber

1 cup peeled, julienned daikon radish

1 bunch cilantro sprigs

2 1-pound Maine lobsters, steamed, shelled, and cut into
　　small pieces

1 bunch green onion* cut into long strips

* Green onion can be classified as a type of scallion. Both can be used interchangeably. True scallions have straight-sided bases. Green onions are usually slightly curved at the base, showing the beginning of a bulb.

1 bunch mint sprigs
1 cup bean sprouts
½ honeydew melon, peeled, seeded, and thinly sliced
12 cabbage leaves, steamed

1. Make a marinade. In a glass bowl mix together seasoned rice vinegar, togarashi, salt, and pepper.

2. Toss cucumber and daikon radish and marinade for 10 minutes.

3. Place side by side on a cutting board the cilantro, lobster meat, green onion, mint, bean sprouts, the marinated daikon and cucumbers, and honeydew melon slices.

4. Blanch the cabbage leaves in salted, boiling water until softened. Place on another cutting board. Pat cabbage leaves dry with a towel.

5. Lay the cabbage leaves flat and trim off the thickest part of the rib.

6. Place 1 to 2 tablespoons cilantro, lobster, green onion, mint, bean sprouts, marinated cucumber and daikon, and honeydew on a cabbage leaf.

7. Partly roll the bottom edge of leaf up to enclose filling. Fold in the leaf sides. Continue rolling up the cabbage leaf. Repeat with the remaining 11 cabbage leaves.

8. Cover and refrigerate.

Tangerine Soy Dipping Sauce
⅓ cup low-sodium soy sauce
¼ cup tangerine juice
¼ cup mirin
3 tablespoons minced scallions
3 tablespoons yuzu juice
2 tablespoons brown rice vinegar
2 tablespoons minced fresh mint
2 tablespoons minced cilantro
1 teaspoon hot chili oil
1 teaspoon grated fresh ginger
½ teaspoon sambal

1. In mixing bowl combine all ingredients. Whisk together. Set aside.

Presentation

2 tablespoons black sesame seeds

2 tablespoons white sesame seeds

12 sprigs fresh chives

12 sprigs cilantro

12 sprigs fresh mint

1. Remove spring rolls from refrigerator. Cut each in half diagonally.

2. For each serving place four pieces of spring roll in the center of chilled sushi plate. Place dipping sauce in a little bowl next to rolls. Sprinkle rolls with black and white sesame seeds.

3. Garnish with bouquet made of two sprigs each of chive, cilantro, and mint sprigs.

NOTE: This is also delicious with your favorite shellfish, ahi tuna, or salmon instead of the lobster).

YIELD: **6 SERVINGS**

Mediterranean Chicken Breast with Aromatic Kidney Beans

Mediterranean Chicken Breast

1 tablespoon extra virgin olive oil

6 8-ounce skinless, boneless chicken breasts

Sea salt and freshly ground black pepper

½ cup tomatoes, peeled, seeded, and finely chopped

12 kalamata olives, pitted and chopped

1 roasted green bell pepper, peeled, seeded, and diced

2 tablespoons minced shallots

1 clove garlic, minced

Juice of 1 lemon

¼ cup chicken stock

Pinch saffron threads

1. Heat olive oil in large heavy skillet over medium heat.

2. Season chicken breasts to taste with salt and pepper.

3. Sear chicken breasts, cooking 2 minutes per side.

4. Add tomatoes, olives, bell pepper, shallots, garlic, and lemon juice. Cook 1 minute.

5. Add chicken stock and saffron. Cover. Cook 3 to 5 minutes, until chicken is cooked through.

6. Remove chicken from skillet, and set aside. Season to taste. Keep warm.

Aromatic Kidney Beans
1 quart chicken stock
½ cup kidney beans, soaked overnight and drained
1 tablespoon extra virgin olive oil
¼ cup diced turkey bacon
½ cup minced Vidalia onion
½ cup finely diced Japanese eggplant
1 stalk celery, finely diced
1 clove garlic, minced
1 tablespoon finely chopped fresh lemon thyme
1 tablespoon finely chopped fresh tarragon
Sea salt
Cayenne pepper

1. Bring chicken stock to boil in large pot. Add kidney beans, and lower heat. Simmer 30 to 45 minutes, until beans are tender. Drain and set aside.

2. Heat olive oil in large saucepan over medium heat. Add turkey bacon. Cook 1 minute.

3. Add onion, eggplant, celery, garlic, lemon thyme, and tarragon. Cook 3 to 5 minutes, without browning.

4. Reduce heat to low. Add beans. Cook 10 minutes. Season to taste with salt, cayenne, and freshly ground black pepper.

Presentation
6 sprigs tarragon
½ cup finely julienned tomato
2 tablespoons finely chopped chives
3 tablespoons extra virgin olive oil

1. For each serving place a mound of kidney beans in the center of a warmed pasta bowl. Top with one chicken breast.

2. Ladle sauce around chicken. Top with tarragon sprig. Garnish with tomato and chives and drizzle with olive oil.

YIELD: **6** SERVINGS

Pistachio Almond–Crusted Wild Striped Bass with Avocado Butter and Fennel-Grapefruit Salad

Pistachio Almond Crust

½ cup unsalted pistachios, shelled

¼ cup sliced almonds, blanched

1 teaspoon curry powder

1 teaspoon ground cumin

½ teaspoon ground white pepper

¼ teaspoon kosher salt

1. Place all ingredients in food processor. Pulse until coarse, about 20 seconds.

2. Set aside.

Wild Striped Bass

6 7-ounce wild striped bass fillets, scaled, skin on, pin bone removed

2 tablespoons extra virgin olive oil

1. Spread pistachio-almond mixture on cookie sheet and coat only flesh side of bass fillets.

2. Heat olive oil in skillet over medium heat. Sauté coated side of bass until golden brown, approximately 1 minute. Flip over. Continue to cook about 4 minutes.

3. Remove fish fillet from skillet. Set aside.

Avocado Butter

2 tablespoons unsalted butter, softened

¾ cup ripe avocado

2 tablespoons chopped fresh cilantro

2 cloves garlic, minced

Juice of 1 lime

Sea salt and freshly ground black pepper

Dash Tabasco

1. In small mixing bowl whip butter until soft and creamy.

2. In separate bowl, blend avocado, cilantro, and garlic. Add lime juice, salt, pepper, and Tabasco.

3. Stir avocado mixture into butter.

Fennel-Grapefruit Salad

1 large fennel bulb, halved

6 medium shiitake mushrooms, stemmed

2 pink grapefruits, cut into segments

2 Belgian endives, cut into 8 lengthwise wedges

1 cup cucumber, peeled, seeded, diced

¼ cup roasted green bell peppers, diced

Juice of 1 lime

2 tablespoons brown rice vinegar

1 tablespoon chopped scallions

1 tablespoon chopped mint

Pinch ground star anise

Pinch cayenne pepper

Sea salt and freshly ground black pepper

1. On hot grill, broil fennel and shiitake mushrooms approximately 2 minutes. Remove from grill.

2. Cut fennel and shiitake mushrooms into thin slices. Set aside. Cool.

3. In a large bowl combine fennel and mushrooms with remaining ingredients. Season to taste with salt and pepper.

Presentation

½ cup arugula sprouts

2 tablespoons pumpkin seed oil

1. For each serving, place a portion of fennel salad in center of a plate. Top with bass fillet.

2. Spoon avocado butter over bass. Garnish with arugula sprouts. Drizzle plate with pumpkin seed oil.

YIELD: **6** SERVINGS

Pan-Seared Organic Sonoma Chicken Breast with Wilted Leeks, Swiss Chard, and Roasted-Tomato Coulis

Pan-Seared Organic Sonoma Chicken Breast

6 8-ounce organic Sonoma chicken breasts, bone in

2 tablespoons extra virgin olive oil

1 teaspoon chopped pineapple sage

1 teaspoon garam masala

Sea salt and freshly ground black pepper

1. Preheat oven to 375°F.

2. On large platter, season chicken with 1 teaspoon olive oil, pineapple sage, garam masala, salt, and pepper. Set aside for 30 minutes.

3. Heat 1 teaspoon olive oil in heavy, ovenproof skillet over moderate heat. Place chicken in skillet, skin side down. Cook until golden. Turn over.

4. Finish in oven. Bake 20 to 25 minutes. Set aside and keep warm.

Wilted Leeks and Swiss Chard

2 tablespoons extra virgin olive oil

3 packed cups chopped red Swiss chard, washed, patted dry

1½ cups leeks, washed, patted dry, thinly sliced on diagonal, white part only

¼ cup thinly chopped shallots

2 cloves garlic, peeled, slivered

¼ cup vegetable stock

Juice of 1 lemon
1 sprig marjoram
Sea salt and freshly ground black pepper
¼ cup heavy cream
1 tablespoon fresh parsley
1 tablespoon chopped chives

1. In saucepan, heat olive oil over moderate heat.

2. Add Swiss chard, leeks, shallots, and garlic. Cook 3 minutes without browning, stirring constantly.

3. Add vegetable stock, lemon juice, marjoram, pinch of salt, and pepper. Reduce liquid to a thick, syrupy consistency.

4. Add heavy cream and parsley. Raise heat to high. Cook approximately 1 minute. Sprinkle with chives.

5. Season to taste with salt and pepper. Keep warm.

Roasted-Tomato Coulis
3 medium tomatoes, cored and quartered
2 tablespoons extra virgin olive oil
1 pinch paprika
1 whole star anise
¼ cup diced white onions
1 clove garlic, crushed
½ cup finely chopped fennel
Sea salt and freshly ground black pepper
Dash Tabasco
¼ cup hazelnut oil
2 tablespoons finely chopped basil

1. In heavy nonstick skillet roast tomatoes at high heat 2 minutes.

2. Lower heat to medium. Add olive oil, paprika, and star anise. Cook 1 minute.

3. Add onions, garlic, fennel, salt, and pepper. Stir well. Cook another 3 minutes without browning.

4. Remove star anise.

5. Pour mixture into blender. Add Tabasco and hazelnut oil. Blend at high speed.

6. Pass through fine sieve. Stir in basil. Season to taste with salt and pepper.

Presentation
12 large asparagus spears, peeled, steamed
6 sprigs pineapple sage

1. For each serving place wilted leek and Swiss chard in center of a warmed plate. Top with chicken breast.

2. Spoon roasted-tomato coulis around plate. Garnish with asparagus and pineapple sage.

YIELD: **6** SERVINGS

Southwestern Spiced Bluefish with Chickpea and Hearts of Palm Salad

Southwestern Spiced Bluefish
¼ cup chopped pecans
¼ cup pumpkin seeds, toasted
½ teaspoon pasilla chili powder
½ teaspoon achiote powder
6 6-ounce bluefish fillets, skinless, pin bone removed
2 tablespoons extra virgin olive oil

1. Preheat oven to 350°F.

2. Combine chopped pecans, pumpkin seeds, chili powder, and achiote powder in food processor. Pulse to a coarse meal. Transfer to a flat plate.

3. Pat fish dry with paper towels. Coat one side of fish fillet with nut-spice mixture.

4. Transfer fish, crust side up, to an oiled baking sheet.

5. Using pastry brush lightly crust with olive oil. Place in oven. Bake 20 minutes.

Chickpea and Hearts of Palm Salad

½ cup chickpeas, soaked overnight, drained

2 hearts of palm, sliced thinly crosswise

2 medium tangerines, peeled, diced (reserve juice)

1 medium clove garlic, crushed

1 medium tomato, peeled, diced (reserve juice)

½ cup diced cucumber

¼ cup minced red onion

¼ cup chopped parsley

3 tablespoons avocado oil

1 tablespoon chopped chives

1 teaspoon chopped lemon verbena

Sea salt and fresh ground black pepper

1. Place chickpeas in large pot. Add water to cover. Bring to boil.

2. Reduce heat. Cover and simmer for 45 minutes or until chickpeas are tender. Drain. Cool to room temperature.

3. Combine remaining ingredients in large bowl. Add cooled chickpeas. Season to taste with salt and pepper. Toss.

Presentation

6 sprigs lemon verbena

2 tablespoons avocado oil

1. For each serving place a portion of chickpea salad in center of a large shallow bowl. Top with bluefish.

2. Garnish with lemon verbena sprig. Drizzle with avocado oil.

YIELD: **6** SERVINGS

Desserts

Oven-Baked Apples

6 large Granny Smith or Fuji apples, cored, unpeeled

⅓ cup sliced almonds, lightly toasted

½ cup boysenberries

1 teaspoon lemon zest

½ teaspoon ground nutmeg

¼ teaspoon ground cardamom

1 tablespoon hazelnut oil

⅔ cup apple cider

3 cinnamon sticks, broken in half

6 tablespoons crème fraîche or whole milk unflavored yogurt

6 sprigs mint

1. Preheat oven to 350°F.

2. Score apples once around middle to prevent bursting. Set apples in shallow 1 to 1½ quart baking dish, just large enough to hold them without touching.

3. In a small bowl, combine almonds, boysenberries, lemon zest, nutmeg, and cardamom.

4. Gently pack mixture into apples. Scatter any remaining filling into pan. Drizzle apples with hazelnut oil. Pour apple cider into pan. Cover apples loosely with aluminum foil to prevent burning. Bake for 20 minutes.

5. Uncover. Baste with juice in bottom of pan.

6. Return apples to oven. Bake until tender but not mushy, about 20 minutes more, basting every 5 minutes.

7. Remove apples from oven.

8. Place juice into saucepan and simmer over low heat until reduced by half.

9. Place each apple in a warmed shallow soup bowl. Spoon reduced juice over apples. Garnish with crème fraîche or yogurt, cinnamon sticks, and mint sprig.

YIELD: **6** SERVINGS

Peach, Cherry, and Blueberry Crumble with Orange-Scented Nut Topping

Orange-Scented Nut Topping
1 cup rolled oats
¼ cup chopped pecans
¼ cup slivered almonds
¼ cup chopped cashews
¼ teaspoon star anise powder
3 tablespoons grapeseed oil
Zest of 1 orange

1. Preheat oven to 375°F.
2. In a medium bowl combine all ingredients. Set aside.

Peaches and Cherries
3 large, ripe peaches, peeled, pitted, and diced
2 pints ripe whole cherries, stemmed and pitted
1 pint blueberries, fresh or frozen
1 tablespoon rose flower water
1 teaspoon almond extract
1 teaspoon vanilla extract
½ cup almond flour

1. In a large bowl combine fruit, rose flower water, and almond and vanilla extracts. Toss gently with large spoon.

2. Sprinkle with almond flour. Toss until fruit is evenly coated.

3. Slide peach and cherry mixture into 13 x 9-inch baking dish. Cover with topping.

4. Place dish on baking sheet. Bake 45 to 60 minutes, until top is browned and juices are bubbling over.

YIELD: 8 TO 12 SERVINGS

Appendix B
Resources

For acne products containing anti-inflammatory/anti-aging ingredients

    N.V. Perricone, M.D., Ltd. (888-823-7837, www.nvperriconemd.com)

    NuSkin

For products to diminish the appearance of scars

    N.V. Perricone, M.D. Cosmeceuticals Alpha Lipoic Acid Face Firming Activator, N.V. Perricone, M.D., Ltd. (888-823-7837, www.nvperriconemd.com)

    ReJuveness Pure Silicone Sheeting (www.rejuveness.com)

Recommended vitamin and nutritional supplements

    Multivitamin packets containing entire Acne Program "Skin-Clear"™, N.V. Perricone, M.D., Ltd. (888-823-7837, www.nvperriconemd.com)

    Sephora

    For more information about a Sephora store in your area, call Sephora's Customer Service at 1-877-SEPHORA.

    Selected Saks Fifth Avenue stores

    For more information about a Saks store in your area, CALL 1-877-551-SAKS

    Nordstrom

    For more information about a Nordstrom store in your area, call 1-888-282-6060

    Selected Neiman Marcus stores

    For more information about a Neiman Marcus store in your area, call 1-888-888-4757

    Optimum Health International

    1-800-228-1507

For vitamins, minerals, nutrients, and amino acids

Bronson Pharmaceuticals (800-235-3200; fax 801-756-5739)
Life Extension Foundation (800-544-4440, www.lef.org)

Yoga information/recommended reading

International Association of Yoga Therapists (www.iayt.org/benefits.
html), Yoga Research and Education Center, International Association of Yoga Therapists, P.O. Box 426, Manton, CA 96059
(530-474-5700, www.yrec.org)

The Yoga of Breath: A Step-by-Step Guide to Pranayama by Richard
Rosen (Boston: Shambhala, 2002).

Wild alaskan salmon and organic blueberries

Vital Choice Seafood 605 30 Street, Anacortes, WA 98221 (800-608-
4825, www.vitalchoice.com)

Seafood recipes

National Seafood Educators, established in 1977, is a good information source for seafood buying, preparation, cooking, and nutrition. Titles in their award-winning cookbook series are *Seafood
Twice a Week, Seafood Grilling Twice a Week, Simple Steps to Cooking
Seafood Twice a Week* and *Wild Alaskan Seafood Twice a Week*. Books
and seafood cooking items may be ordered by calling 800-348-
0010.

Pomegranate Juice and Pomegranate Extract

For nutrition information and stores in your area that carry Pom-
Wonderful visit www.pomwonderful.com.

Anti-oxidant Rich Teas

YH Tea Company, San Francisco, California, www.yhteas.com,
peter@yhteas.com, 415-395-0868

Appendix C
GLOSSARY

ACCUTANE (13-CIS-RETINOIC ACID): effective prescription treatment for severe (i.e., cystic or nodular) acne but with possible serious side effects.

ACETYLCHOLINE: a derivative of choline that is released at the ends of nerve fibers and is involved in the transmission of nerve impulses in the body, including impulses that cause muscles to contract.

ACNE: a systemic inflammatory disease characterized by skin eruptions.

ACNE LESIONS (PIMPLES, BLACKHEADS, WHITEHEADS): acne lesions are categorized in five grades. Grade 1 includes miniscule microcomedones and the more easily noticeable comedones (whiteheads and blackheads traditionally but erroneously referred to as "noninflammatory" acne lesions). Grade 2 lesions are papules—the small, pink, visibly inflamed bumps that are tender to the touch, and which conventional science recognizes as inflammatory. Grade 3 acne lesions are pustules—lesions with more visible inflammation than papules. Grade 4 acne lesions are nodules—large, painful, solid lesions extending deep into the skin accompanied by visible inflammation. Grade 5 acne lesions are cysts—inflamed, pus-filled lesions extending deep into the skin. This occurs when several nodules merge resulting in a giant lesion.

ADRENAL HORMONES: cortisol, DHEA, and adrenaline are the three adrenal stress hormones.

ALPHA HYDROXY ACIDS: natural exfoliating acids derived from fruit, milk, and sugar cane that have anti-inflammatory properties.

ALPHA LIPOIC ACID (THIOTIC ACID): the "universal antioxidant," alpha lipoic acid is both water and fat soluble, a characteristic that gives it the unique ability to reach all portions of the cell, providing superior protection from free radical damage and inflammation. It also helps restore the antioxidant powers of vitamins C and E after they have been depleted.

AMINO ACIDS: molecules that the body uses to make proteins. Eight dietary amino acids are essential to human life.

ANDROGENS (ANDROGENIC HORMONES): steroidal hormones, such as testosterone or androsterone, that control the development and maintenance of masculine characteristics. Androgens occur naturally in both sexes and tend to stimulate oil production in the skin by binding to a special receptor on the oil gland. A special enzyme present in the oil gland converts androgens, such as testosterone, into a more powerful acne-promoting androgen called dihydrotestosterone (DHT).

ANTI-INFLAMMATORIES: chemical substances that tend to reduce inflammation in the body.

ANTIOXIDANTS: substances that prevent or reverse the development of free radicals.

AP-1: a transcription factor activated in many ways, one of which is sunlight, that promotes the secretion of a collagen-digesting enzyme called metalloproteinase.

ARACHIDONIC ACID: an unsaturated fatty acid found in animal fats that is essential in human nutrition and is a precursor in the biosynthesis of certain prostaglandins. Arachidonic acid is produced by cells in response to the presence of free radicals and typically triggers a cascade of inflammatory reactions. Limiting intake of foods high in saturated fats (red meat, cheese, etc.) that convert to arachidonic acid can help reduce inflammation.

ASCORBYL PALMITATE: fat-soluble form of vitamin C; also known as vitamin C ester.

ATPASE: enzyme that hydrolyzes ATP and is therefore essential to efficient energy production in body cells.

ATROPHIC SCARS: deep, indented scars resulting from collagen loss.

AUTONOMIC NERVOUS SYSTEM: the network of nerves governing functions such as blood pressure, heart rate, bowel and bladder emptying, and digestion.

BASAL LAYER: the bottom layer of the epidermis that produces new skin cells.

BENZOYL PEROXIDE: popular acne medication that is available both in over-the-counter and through prescription. Its effectiveness comes from its antibacterial acne medication that also acts as a peeling agent and may limit the secretion of certain oils that contain fatty acids, which contribute to acne flare-ups.

BLACKHEAD (see OPEN COMEDO): a dark acne lesion consisting of a plug of keratin and sebum. Only a physician should extract plugs, since damage to the surrounding tissues occasioned by squeezing can lead to scarring. Contrary to conventional medical belief, blackheads are characterized by inflammation.

CATECHINS: antioxidant polyphenols from plants that help stabilize collagen and prevent capillary fragility.

CATECHOLAMINES: neurotransmitters and hormones; examples include epinephrine, norepinephrine, and dopamine.

CELL PLASMA MEMBRANE: outer layer of a cell made up of phospholipids that is susceptible to free radical damage.

CHOLESTEROL: white crystalline substance found in animal tissues and various foods that is also made by the liver and is a key constituent of cell membranes and precursor to steroid hormones. Its level, form, and oxidation status in the bloodstream can influence the development of arterial plaque and coronary artery disease.

CHOLINESTERASE: one of many enzymes needed for the proper functioning of the nervous system; it breaks down a neurotransmitter called acetylcholine into its precursors.

CLINDAMYCIN: an antibiotic drug used to treat acne and bacterial infections.

CLOSED COMEDO (WHITEHEAD): a small, firm, pearly-white acne lesion caused by retention of keratin in a sebaceus gland duct that has been blocked by a thin layer of skin cells. Contrary to conventional medical belief, whiteheads are characterized by inflammation. Any attempt to eliminate whiteheads by squeezing or picking can aggravate the inflammatory process.

COLLAGEN: the protein fibers that give the skin strength and flexibility.

COLLAGENASE: enzyme produced by the cells in response to free radicals that damages collagen fibers, creating microscarring that leads to wrinkles.

COMEDO (plural COMEDONES): a plug of keratin and sebum, blackened at the surface, within a follicle.

COMEDOGENIC AGENTS: ingredients in cosmetics that tend to clog pores and cause or promote comedones (acne lesions).

CORTISOL: an adrenal hormone released in response to physical and emotional stresses, including lack of sleep. Among other destructive bodily effects, cortisol can stimulate acne flare-ups by raising blood sugar levels, promoting inflammation, and stimulating the skin's sebaceous glands.

CRYOTHERAPY: therapeutic freezing of acne lesions with dry ice or liquid nitrogen.

CYST: an abnormal membranous sac containing a gaseous, liquid, or semisolid substance.

CYTOKINES: messenger peptides produced by lymphocytes (white blood cells) in response to free radicals and other agents. Many, but not all, are inflammatory.

CYTOSOL: the watery interior of the cell.

DERMIS: the lower layer of the skin that contains nerve endings, sweat glands, and collagen and elastin fibers.

DESQUAMATION: the natural process by which a keratinocyte (skin cell) gradually migrates to the surface and is sloughed off.

DHEA (DEHYDROEPIANDROSTERONE): male steroid hormone secreted by the adrenal glands and, to a lesser extent, by the ovaries and testes. The body can convert DHEA into testosterone and estrogen.

DHT (DIHYDROTESTOSTERONE): powerful acne-promoting androgen the body makes from testosterone.

DMAE (DIMETHYLAMINOETHANOL): antioxidant membrane stabilizer that is a precursor to acetylcholine. DMAE can act as a cognitive enhancer, a smoothing, anti-aging, muscle-toning facial topical and a therapeutic aid for acne scarring.

EEG (ELECTROENCEPHALOGRAM): test measuring brain wave activity.

ELASTIN FIBERS: protein fibers that, along with collagen, are responsible for the strength, elasticity, and texture of the skin.

EMG (ELECTROMYOGRAM): test measuring nerve transmission to muscles.

EMOLLIENT: agent (typically a moisturizer) that softens or soothes the skin.

ENDOCRINE SYSTEM: bodily system that produces hormones and

other chemicals that regulate key bodily functions, consisting of the endocrine glands, which include the pituitary, thyroid, parathyroid, and adrenal glands, as well as the islets of Langerhans, the ovaries, and the testes.

ENZYMES: bodily protein that enables vital chemical reactions in the body.

EPIDERMIS: outer layer of the skin.

EPITHELIAL TISSUES: skin and the mucous membranes lining the internal body surfaces.

ERYTHROMYCIN: antibiotic drug used to treat acne and bacterial infections.

ESSENTIAL FATTY ACIDS (EFAs): two types of fatty acids are essential to human health, omega-3 and omega-6. As key structural components of cell membranes, EFAs bar foreign molecules, viruses, yeasts, fungi, and bacteria from entering cells, and they help to control the flow of chemical compounds in and out of cells. One EFA is the omega-6 fatty acid called linoleic acid (LA), which is abundant in common cooking oils like safflower, sunflower, and corn oils. The second EFA is an omega-3 fatty acid called alpha-linolenic acid or LNA, which is found in flax- and hemp seed oils. In the absence of dietary LNA the body can substitute either of two other omega-3 EFAs: eicosapentaenoic acid (EPA) and docosahexaenoic acid (DHA), which are found in fatty fish such as salmon, herring, and mackerel. In fact, EPA and DHA are more readily usable by the body, compared to LNA, and offer special benefits to the brain, eyes, and heart. The ideal dietary ratio of omega-6 to omega-3 is 2 to 1, but the omega-6 to omega-3 ratio of the average American diet is closer to 30 to 1.

ESTER: chemical compound that combines an acid and an alcohol. Ascorbyl palmitate—the best known ester of vitamin C—is made by adding a fatty acid from palm oil to L-ascorbic acid.

ESTROGENS: "female" hormones that actually occur naturally in both sexes.

EXFOLIATION: peeling of the outer layer of the skin, typically by use of a mildly abrasive material; or the natural process by which a skin cell gradually migrates to the surface and is sloughed off.

FIBROBLASTS: cells that produce collagen and elastin.

FLAVONOIDS: phytochemicals (plant-based chemicals) with strong antioxidant properties.

FLAXSEED: along with hemp seed and fatty fish such as salmon, this tasty seed is one of the richest sources of omega-3 essential fatty acids (LNA in particular). Flaxseed also contains calcium, iron, niacin, phosphorous, vitamin E, and beneficial lignans—a class of estrogen-like plant compounds that act as antioxidants and may prevent the development of some cancers. Flaxseed has a mild, nutty flavor, and is delicious in yogurt, hot cereal, grain dishes, or stir-fries.

FOLLICLE: a minute depression in the skin, such as those from which hair emerges.

FREE RADICALS: unstable molecules that produce inflammation and promote aging and disease.

GALVANIC SKIN RESPONSE: change in the ability of the skin to conduct electricity, typically caused by an emotional stimulus such as fright.

GAMMA LINOLEIC ACID: anti-inflammatory omega-6 series essential fatty acid found in borage and primrose seed oils.

GLUTATHIONE PEROXIDASE: enzyme that is essential for the removal of toxins produced by lipid metabolism.

GLYCEMIC INDEX: scale that rates foods from one to 100 according to their impact on blood sugar levels.

HDL CHOLESTEROL: cholesterol and triglycerides combine with proteins to form lipoproteins. High density lipoprotein, the so-called good cholesterol, removes excess cholesterol from arterial blood and arterial walls and disposes of it before it can do any damage. In fact, it is the lipoprotein that is good, not the cholesterol it carries.

HEMATOCRIT: the percent of whole blood comprised of red blood cells.

HEMOGLOBIN: the main component of red blood cells; a protein that carries oxygen away from the lungs and carbon dioxide back to the lungs.

HGH (HUMAN GROWTH HORMONE): hormone secreted by the pituitary gland. Declining levels as we age are linked to weight gain, sagging skin, and lower energy levels.

HOMOCYSTEINE: amino acid used in cellular metabolism and to make proteins. High concentrations in the blood may increase the risk of heart disease by damaging the lining of blood vessels and promoting blood clotting.

HYDROXYL FREE RADICAL: particularly dangerous type of free radical.

HYDROXYTYROSOL: polyphenol antioxidant found in extra virgin olive oil.

HYPERTROPHIC SCAR: enlarged, raised scar, made up of an excess of collagen that develops during healing.

INDOLES: powerful anticancer compounds found in cabbage, brussels sprouts, cauliflower, and kale.

INDUCIBLE NITRIC OXIDE: a metabolic end product that causes smooth muscle to relax.

INFLAMMATION: a biochemical response to injury or infection ranging from the invisible cellular level to the visible, characterized by pain, redness, swelling, and sometimes loss of function. Inflammation can also be produced throughout the body by an excess of free radicals stemming from dietary factors such as sugars and other proinflammatory foods which leads to aging and age-related diseases.

INTERLEUKINS: various proteins produced by immune system cells (lymphocytes, macrophages, and monocytes) that help regulate cell-mediated immunity. Many are proinflammatory.

KELOID: a red, raised formation of fibrous scar tissue caused by excessive tissue repair in response to trauma or infection.

KERATIN: the protein that is the primary constituent of hair, nails, and skin.

KERATINIZATION: the process of maturation of basal skin cells as they move toward the surface of the skin and become the stratum corneum.

KERATINOCYTES: component of the outermost layer of skin; cells containing keratin, a protein, that provides a durable mechanical and moisture barrier to protect underlying tissues.

LASER LIGHT THERAPY: treatment of acne with a specific wavelength of light that destroys the *Propionibacterium acnes*.

LDL CHOLESTEROL: low density lipoprotein cholesterol, or so-called bad cholesterol, can accumulate in artery walls and become oxidized, thus causing atherosclerosis.

LESION: wounded or infected area of skin.

LEUKOTRIENE: compound produced by the arachidonic acid cascade that prompts proinflammatory changes throughout the body.

LYCOPENE: antioxidant carotene compound found in tomatoes.

LYMPHOCYTE: the type of white blood cell that plays key roles in immune responses to foreign bodies (microbes, toxins).

MELANIN: pigment found in human skin.

MELANOCYTE: cell in the skin that produces and contains the pigment melanin.

MICROCOMEDO: first and smallest type of acne lesion that occurs at the earliest stages when the follicle walls are just beginning to be stretched by trapped sebum. Microcomedones cannot be seen without a microscope.

MITOCHONDRIA: the vital, energy-producing organelles within the cells.

N-ACETYL CYSTEINE: modified form of the amino acid cysteine that helps the body synthesize glutathione—an important anti-inflammatory agent and antioxidant.

NEUROPEPTIDES: short-chain peptides, such as endorphins, found in brain tissue but also found in many other cells of the body including skin cells.

NF-K B (NUCLEAR FACTOR KAPPA B): genetic transcription factor triggered by oxidative stress that in turn promotes production of highly inflammatory messenger chemicals (cytokines) known as interleukins.

NODULE: small mass of tissue or grouping of cells.

NONCOMEDOGENIC: not pore clogging.

OLEIC ACID: monounsaturated fatty acid found in olive oil and peanuts that helps omega-3 oil pass into the cell membrane.

OMEGA-3 FATTY ACID: anti-inflammatory essential fatty acid found in fish, oatmeal, nuts, and soy products.

OPEN COMEDO (BLACKHEAD): dark-colored acne lesion consisting of a plug of keratin and sebum. The dark color derives from melanin (skin pigment), not dirt. Contrary to conventional medical belief, blackheads are characterized by inflammation. Any attempt to eliminate blackheads by squeezing or picking can aggravate the inflammatory process.

OXIDATION: process by which the positive charge or valence of (an element) is increased by removing electrons. Oxidation of cellular materials by free radicals is generally damaging.

OXIDATIVE STRESS: highly oxidized environment within cells, where there is an excess of free radicals and a lack of antioxidants, which always leads to inflammation.

PANTOTHENIC ACID: B vitamin that forms part of a molecule known as coenzyme A, which is essential for energy production in the body. Pantothenic acid is concentrated in the adrenal glands where it is necessary for the production of hormones, including sex hormones. A powerful antioxidant and anti-inflammatory, pantothenic acid also blocks the oxidation of important fats in cells.

PAPULE: a small, solid, usually inflammatory lesion of the skin that does not contain pus.

PHENOLS (POLYPHENOLS or PHENOLICS): powerful antioxidants found in tea, chocolate, red wine, grape juice, and many herbs and vegetables. Phenols fight inflammation and cell damage that leads to chronic conditions such as cancer and heart diseases. Special phenols in tea called catechins appear to aid in weight control.

PHOSPHATIDYL CHOLINE: compound found naturally in lecithin that offers important protection to the cell plasma membrane.

PHOSPHOLIPIDS: any of various phosphorous-containing lipids—such as lecithin and cephalin—that are composed mainly of fatty acids, a phosphate group, and a simple organic molecule. Phospholipids are found in all living cells and in the bilayers of cell plasma membranes.

POLYMORPHONUCLEAR CELLS: white blood cells that fight bacterial infections by engulfing and digesting bacteria. They form pus and are the chief constituents of abscesses.

PROANTHROCYANIDINS (OPCs OR PYCNOGENOLS): strong antioxidants found in pine needles, grapes, and berries that stabilize collagen and boost the antioxidant properties of vitamins E and C.

PROINFLAMMATORY: promoting inflammation.

PROPIONIBACTERIUM ACNES: bacterium, commonly found in the sebaceous glands of human skin, that releases lipases (fat-digesting enzymes) to digest sebum. The combination of digestive byproducts (fatty acids) and bacterial antigens (irritants) stimulates an intense local inflammation that ruptures the follicle. A lesion then forms on the surface of the skin in the form of a pustule.

PROSTAGLANDINS: group of short-lived but potent hormone-like substances produced in human tissues from arachidonic acid. Prostaglandins mediate a wide range of physiological functions, such as control of blood pressure, contraction of smooth muscle, and modulation of inflammation. Some are proinflammatory, while others are anti-inflammatory.

PUSTULE (PIMPLE): a small swelling.

QUERCETIN: antioxidant bioflavonoid found in red wine, tea, onions, apples, and other foods.

RADIO WAVE THERAPY: acne therapy in which the surface of the skin is heated with radio waves after being cooled with liquid nitrogen.

REDOX (REDUCTION-OXIDATION) LEVEL: ratio of free radicals to antioxidants in a cell.

RETENTION HYPERKERATOSIS: excessive build-up of skin cells in follicles. These dead skin cells combine with oil in the follicle to create a plug that traps acne-promoting bacteria. Retention hyperkeratosis is triggered by inflammation and mediated by cytokines such as interleukin-1.

RETIN-A (TRETINOIN, 13-CIS-RETINOIC ACID, or RETIN-A ACID): acidic form of vitamin A, active in skin. When applied topically, it normalizes the desquamation inside the follicle, helping to loosen clogs. Retin-A promotes inflammation. Retinol, the alcohol form of vitamin A, is used in cosmetics because it is converted into the skin to small amounts of Retin-A.

RETINOIDS: natural or synthetic derivatives of vitamin A.

ROSACEA: chronic inflammation of the nose, chin, or forehead, characterized by redness or acnelike eruptions.

SATURATED FAT: fatty acid that increases the risk of heart disease; found primarily in animal fats such as butter, beef, and pork.

SEBACEOUS GLAND: skin gland that produces sebum, the fatty substance, which, under the right circumstances, can help clog pores and produce acne.

SEBUM: the semifluid secretion of the sebaceous glands, consisting chiefly of fat, keratin, and cellular material.

SECRETAGOGUE: hormonal or dietary substance that increases specific chemical secretions from cells.

SOMATIC: of or affecting the body.

SPIN TRAPS: a technique for detecting free radicals in living organisms.

SPIRONOLACTONE: diuretic medication that binds to the body's androgen receptors, thereby preventing the conversion of testosterone to the more powerful hormone DHT.

STRATUM CORNEUM: the topmost layer of the epidermis, made of dead, flat skin cells that shed about every two weeks.

SUBCUTANEOUS: located just beneath the skin.

SUPEROXIDISMUTASE (SOD): antioxidant produced by the body in response to the presence of free radicals.

TEMPEH: a fermented, high-protein soybean food suitable for stir-frying and use in casseroles, etc.

TESTOSTERONE: steroid hormone produced primarily in the testes but also in small quantities in the ovaries, adrenal glands, and placenta. Testosterone production is stimulated in part by high blood levels of insulin, which rise in response to excessive dietary sugars. The sebaceous glands produce more sebum in response to high levels of testosterone, and acne is promoted by an overabundance of sebum. Thus, testosterone tends to promote acne.

TETRACYCLINE: antibiotic drug used to treat acne and bacterial infections.

THYROXIN: iodine-containing thyroid hormone that increases the rate of cell metabolism and regulates growth; made synthetically for the treatment of thyroid disorders.

TOCOPHEROLS: group of closely related fat-soluble, antioxidant phenol compounds constituting vitamin E and similar antioxidants.

TOCOTRIENOL: type of vitamin E compound. Tocopherols are the type of vitamin E compound commonly used in vitamin E supplements. However, when vitamin E is tested in an environment that mimics the cell plasma membrane, the tocotrienol portion exerts 40 times more antioxidant potential than alpha-tocopherol. Research indicates that tocotrienols penetrate rapidly through skin to efficiently combat oxidative stress induced by UV or ozone, and that tocotrienols are the portion of dietary vitamin E that mammals accumulate preferentially in skin.

TOFU: high-protein soybean curds that are also rich in calcium.

TRANSCRIPTION FACTORS: proteins that bind to DNA and play a role in the regulation of gene expression by promoting gene transcription—a process in which one DNA strand is used as template to synthesize a complementary strip of RNA. "Gene expression" means the production of a protein or a functional piece of RNA from its gene.

TRIGLYCERIDES: lipids (fatty compounds) that circulate in the blood to transport and store fats. High triglyceride levels accompanied by low HDL levels are associated with high risk of arteriosclerosis and cardiovascular disease.

TUMOR NECROSIS FACTOR (TNF): inflammatory immune system compound that can inhibit tumor growth but can also cause damage to healthy cells.

VLDL CHOLESTEROL: very low density lipoprotein cholesterol is considered the worst form of cholesterol, in terms of promoting atherosclerosis.

WHITEHEAD (CLOSED COMEDO): A small, firm, pearly, white acne bump caused by retention of keratin (skin protein) in an oil gland duct that has been blocked by a thin layer of epithelium (skin cells). Contrary to conventional medical belief, whiteheads are characterized by inflammation.

References

Chapter 1

1. Jeanne Achterberg. *Woman as Healer* (Boston: Shambala Publications, Inc., 1990), pp. 110–11.
2. E. Ingham, E. A. Eady, C. E. Goodwin, J. H. Cove, and W. J. Cunliffe, "Proinflammatory Levels of Interleukin-1 Alpha-like Bioactivity Are Present in the Majority of Open Comedones in Acne Vulgaris," *Journal of Investigative Dermatology* 98 (1992): 895–901.

Chapter 2

1. C. C. Zouboulis, "Is Acne Vulgaris a Genuine Inflammatory Disease?" *Dermatology* 203 (2001): 277–79.
2. N. Hjorth, "Traditional Topical Treatment of Acne," *Acta Dermatology Venereology* 89 supplement (1980): 53–56.
3. N. Egan, M. C. Loesche, and M. M. Baker, "Randomized, Controlled, Bilateral (Split-Face) Comparison Trial of the Tolerability and Patient Preference of Adapalene Gel 0.1% and Tretinoin Microsphere Gel 0.1% for the Treatment of Acne Vulgaris," *Cutis* 68 supplement (October 2001): 20–24.
4. M. Schaller, R. Steinle, and H. C. Korting, "Light and Electron Microscopic Findings in Human Epidermis Reconstructed in Vitro Upon Topical Application of Liposomal Tretinoin," *Acta Dermatology Venereology* 77 (March 1997): 122–26.

Chapter 3

1. J. C. Shaw, "Acne: Effect of Hormones on Pathogenesis and Management," *American Journal of Clinical Dermatology* 3 (2002): 571–78.
2. A. Lemay and Y. Poulin, "Oral Contraceptives as Anti-Androgenic Treatment of Acne," *Journal of Obstetrics and Gynaecology Canada* 24 (July 2002): 559–67.
3. M. Toyoda and M. Morohashi, "New Aspects in Acne Inflammation," *Dermatology* 206 (2003): 17–23.
4. R. Rosmond, "Stress Induced Disturbances of the HPA Axis: A Pathway to Type 2 Diabetes?" *Medical Science Monitor* 9 (February 2003): RA35–39.
5. A. L. Lee, W. O. Ogle, and R. M. Sapolsky, "Stress and Depression: Possible Links to Neuron Death in the Hippocampus," *Bipolar Disorders* 4 (April 2002): 117–28.

6. R. Nass and M. O. Thorner, "Impact of the GH-Cortisol Ratio on the Age-Dependent Changes in Body Composition," *Growth Hormone & IGF Research* 12 (June 2002): 147–61.

7. A. Polleri, M. V. Gianelli, and G. Murialdo, "Dementia: A Neuroendocrine Perspective," *Journal of Endocrinological Investigation* 25 (January 2002): 73–83.

8. D. B. Corry and M. L. Tuck, "Selective Aspects of the Insulin Resistance Syndrome," *Current Opinion in Nephrology and Hypertension* 10 (July 2001): 507–14.

9. O. M. Wolkowitz, E. S. Epel, and V. I. Reus, "Stress Hormone-Related Psychopathology: Pathophysiological and Treatment Implications," *World Journal of Biological Psychiatry* 2 (July 2001):115–43.

10. K. G. Walton, N. D. Pugh, P. Gelderloos, and P. Macrae, "Stress Reduction and Preventing Hypertension: Preliminary Support for a Psychoneuroendocrine Mechanism," *Journal of Alternative and Complementary Medicine* 1 (1995): 263–83.

11. T. Kakuda, "Neuroprotective Effects of the Green Tea Components Theanine and Catechins," *Biological Pharmacology Bulletin* 25 (December 2002): 1513–18.

12. N. Sueoka, M. Suganuma, E. Sueoka, S. Okabe, S. Matsuyama, K. Imai, K. Nakachi, and H. Fujiki, "A New Function of Green Tea: Prevention of Lifestyle-Related Diseases," *Annals of the New York Academy of Sciences* 928 (April 2001): 274–80.

13. S. J. Bell and G. K. Goodrick, "A Functional Food Product for the Management of Weight," *Critical Reviews in Food Science and Nutrition* 42 (March 2002): 163–78.

14. P. Chantre and D. Lairon, "Recent Findings of Green Tea Extract AR25 (Exolise) and Its Activity for the Treatment of Obesity," *Phytomedicine* 9 (January 2002): 3–8.

15. P. M. Kris-Etherton, K. D. Hecker, A. Bonanome, S. M. Coval, A. E. Binkoski, K. F. Hilpert, A. E. Griel, and T. D. Etherton, "Bioactive Compounds in Foods: Their Role in the Prevention of Cardiovascular Disease and Cancer," *American Journal of Medicine* 113 supplement 9B (December 2002): 71S–88S.

16. J. H. Weisburger, "Chemopreventive Effects of Cocoa Polyphenols on Chronic Diseases," *Experimental Biology and Medicine* 226 (November 2001): 891–97.

17. C. L. Keen, "Chocolate: Food as Medicine/Medicine as Food," *Journal of American College Nutrition* 20 supplement (October 2001): 436S–39S; discussion 440S–42S.

18. Z. D. Draelos, "Cosmetics in Acne and Rosacea," *Seminars in Cutaneous Medicine and Surgery* 20 (September 2001): 209–14.

Chapter 4

1. Y. Lin, M. W. Rajala, J. P. Berger, D. E. Moller, N. Barzilai, and P. E. Scherer, "Hyperglycemia-Induced Production of Acute Phase Reactants in Adipose Tissue," *Journal of Biological Chemistry* 276 (November 9, 2001): 42077–83.

2. K. Tamakoshi, H. Yatsuya, T. Kondo, Y. Hori, M. Ishikawa, H. Zhang, C. Murata, R. Otsuka, S. Zhu, and H. Toyoshima, "The Metabolic Syndrome Is Associated with Elevated Circulating C-Reactive Protein in Healthy Reference Range, A Systemic Low-Grade Inflammatory State," *International Journal of Obesity and Related Metabolic Disorders* 27 (April 2003): 443–49.

3. P. C. Calder, "Dietary Modification of Inflammation with Lipids," *Proceedings of the Nutrition Society* 61 (August 2002): 345–58.

4. G. Casadesus, B. Shukitt–Hale, and J. A. Joseph, "Qualitative versus Quantitative Caloric Intake: Are They Equivalent Paths to Successful Aging?" *Neurobiology of Aging* 23 (September–October 2002): 747–69.

5. R. L. Galli, B. Shukitt-Hale, K. A. Youdim, and J. A. Joseph, "Fruit Polyphenolics and Brain Aging: Nutritional Interventions Targeting Age-Related Neuronal and Behavioral Deficits," *Annals of the New York Academy of Sciences* 959 (April 2002): 128–32.

6. G. Mojzisova and M. Kuchta, "Dietary Flavonoids and Risk of Coronary Heart Disease," *Physiological Research* 50 (2001): 529–35.

7. N. V. Perricone, "Aging: Prevention and Intervention Part I: Antioxidants," *Journal of Geriatric Dermatology* 5 (1997): 1–2.

8. Soon-Mi Shim and Charles R. Santerre, Ph.D., table: "Fatty Acid Content of Farmed and Wild Fish," Department of Foods and Nutrition; Purdue University; 700 W. State St., West Lafayette, IN 47907–2059, available at http://fn.cfs.purdue.edu/anglingindiana/AquaculturevsWildFish/FattyAcidsFarm.pdf

9. G. Mamalakis, M. Tornaritis, and A. Kafatos, "Depression and Adipose Essential Polyunsaturated Fatty Acids," *Prostaglandins, Leukotrienes, and Essential Fatty Acids* 67 (November 2002): 311–18.

10. A. L. Stoll, W. E. Severus, M. P. Freeman, S. Rueter, H. A. Zboyan, E. Diamond, K. K. Cress, L. B. Marangell, "Omega 3 fatty acids in bipolar disorder: a preliminary double-blind, placebo-controlled trial," *Archives of General Psychiatry* 56 (May 1999): 407–12.

B. Nemets, Z. Stahl, R. H. Belmaker, "Addition of Omega-3 Fatty Acid to Maintenance Medication Treatment for Recurrent Unipolar Depressive Disorder," *Am J Psychiatry* (March 2002): 477–9.

11. R. W. Owen, A. Giacosa, W. E. Hull, R. Haubner, G. Wurtele, B. Spiegelhalder, and H. R Bartsch, "Olive-Oil Consumption and Health: The Possible Role of Antioxidants," *Lancet Oncology* 1 (October 2000): 107–12.

12. R. W. Owen, A. Giacosa, W. E. Hull, R. Haubner, B. Spiegelhalder, and H. Bartsch, "The Antioxidant/Anticancer Potential of Phenolic Compounds Isolated from Olive Oil," *European Journal of Cancer Care* 36 (June 2000): 1235–47.

13. ibid.

14. Christos C. Zouboulis, "Is Acne Vulgaris a Genuine Inflammatory Disease?" *Dermatology* 203 (2001): 277–79.

15. L. Cordain, S. Lindeberg, M. Hurtado, K. Hill, S. B. Eaton, and J. Brand-Miller, "Acne Vulgaris: A Disease of Western Civilization," *Archives of Dermatology* 138 (December 2002): 1584–90.

16. H. S. Antilla, S. Reitamo, and J-H. Saurat, "Interleukin 1 Immunoreactivity in Sebaceous Glands," *British Journal of Dermatology* 127 (1992): 585–88.

17. K. D. Boehm, J. K. Yun, K. P. Strohl, and C. A. Elmets, "Messenger RNAs for the Multifunctional Cytokines Interleukin-1 Alpha, Interleukin-1 Beta and Tumor Necrosis Factor-Alpha Are Present in Adnexal Tissues and in Dermis of Normal Human Skin," *Experimental Dermatology* 4 (1995): 335–41.

Chapter 5

1. A. Bierhaus, S. Chevion, M. Chevion, M. Hofmann, P. Quehenberger, T. Illmer, T. Luther, E. Berentshtein, H. Tritschler, M. Muller, P. Wahl, R. Ziegler, and P. P. Nawroth, "Advanced Glycation End Product-Induced Activation of NF-kappa B Is Suppressed by Alpha-Lipoic Acid in Cultured Endothelial Cells," *Diabetes* 46 (September 1997): 1481–90.

2. J. Fuchs and R. Milbradt, "Antioxidant Inhibition of Skin Inflammation Induced by Reactive Oxidants: Evaluation of the Redox Couple Dihydrolipoate/Lipoate," *Skin Pharmacology* 7 (1994): 278–84.

3. V. E. Kagan, A. Shvedova, E. Serbinova, S. Khan, C. Swanson, R. Powell, and L. Packer, "Dihydrolipoic Acid—A Universal Antioxidant Both in the Membrane and in the Aqueous Phase. Reduction of Peroxyl, Ascorbyl and Chromanoxyl Radicals," *Biochemical Pharmacology* 44 (October 20, 1992): 1637–49.

4. Y. J. Suzuki, M. Mizuno, H. J. Tritschler, and L. Packer, "Redox Regulation of NF-kappa B DNA Binding Activity by Dihydrolipoate," *Biochemistry and Molecular Biology International* 36 (June 1995): 241–46.

5. M. Meyer, R. Schreck, and P. A. Baeuerle, "H_2O_2 and Antioxidants Have Opposite Effects on Activation of NF-kappa B and AP-1 in Intact Cells: AP-1 as Secondary Antioxidant-Responsive Factor," *EMBO Journal* 12 (May 1993): 2005–15.

6. T. Ookawara, N. Kawamura, Y. Kitagawa, and N. Taniguchi, "Site-Specific and Random Fragmentation of Cu,Zn-Superoxide Dismutase by Glycation Reaction. Implication of Reactive Oxygen Species," *Journal of Biological Chemistry* 267 (September 15, 1992): 18505–10.

7. E. Naruta and V. Buko, "Hypolipidemic Effect of Pantothenic Acid Derivatives in Mice with Hypothalamic Obesity Induced by Aurothioglucose," *Experimental and Toxicologic Pathology* 53 (October 2001): 393–98.

8. D. G. Genecov, M. Kremer, Sarah Goldberg, and Joshua Cho, "Alpha Lipoic Acid (ALA) and Scar Formation in Repaired Cleft Lips," *Transactions of the 9th International Congress on Cleft Palate and Related Craniofacial Anomalies,* Goteborg, Sweden, 25–29 June, 2001, pp. 495–99.

9. U. N. Das, E. J. Ramos, and M. M. Meguid, "Metabolic Alterations During Inflammation and Its Modulation by Central Actions of Omega-3 Fatty Acids," *Current Opinion in Clinical Nutrition and Metabolic Care* 6 (July 2003): 413–19.

10. A. P. Simopoulos, "Omega-3 Fatty Acids in Inflammation and Autoimmune Diseases," *Journal of the American College of Nutrition* 21 (December 2002): 495–505.

11. H. Seltmann, S. Hornemann, C. E. Orfanos, and C. C. Zouboulis, "Linoleic Acid Induces Accumulation of Neutral Lipids in Undifferentiated Human Sebocytes and Reduces Spontaneous IL-8 Secretion," *Archives for Dermatological Research* 291 (1999): 181.

12. H. Akamatsu and T. Horio, "The Possible Role of Reactive Oxygen Species Generated by Neutrophils in Mediating Acne Inflammation," *Dermatology* 196 (1998): 82–85.

13. D. T. Downing, M. E. Stewart, P. W. Wertz, and J. S. Strauss, "Essential Fatty Acids and Acne," *Journal of the American Academy of Dermatology* 14 (February 1986): 221–25.

14. D. Yam, G. Bott-Kanner, I. Genin, M. Shinitzky, and E. Klainman, (The Effect of Omega-3 Fatty Acids on Risk Factors for Cardiovascular Diseases), *Harefuah* 140 (December 2001): 1156–58, 1230.

15. P. Simoncikova, S. Wein, D. Gasperikova, J. Ukropec, M. Certik, I. Klimes, and E. Sebokova, "Comparison of the Extrapancreatic Action of Gamma-Linolenic Acid and n-3 PUFAs in the High Fat Diet-Induced Insulin Resistance," *Endocrine Regulations* 36 (December 2002): 143–49.

16. Y. Suresh and U. N. Das, "Long-Chain Polyunsaturated Fatty Acids and Chemically Induced Diabetes Mellitus. Effect of Omega-3 Fatty Acids," *Nutrition* 19 (March 2003): 213–28.

17. G. Krey, O. Braissant, F. L'Horset, E. Kalkhoven, M. Perroud, M. G. Parker, and W. Wahli, "Fatty Acids, Eicosanoids, and Hypolipidemic Agents Identified as Ligands of Peroxisome Proliferator-Activated Receptors by Coactivator-Dependent Receptor Ligand Assay," *Molecular Endocrinology* 11 (June 1997): 779–91.

18. C. S. Johnston and B. Luo, "Comparison of the Absorption and Excretion of Three Commercially Available Sources of Vitamin C," *Journal of the American Dietetic Association* 94 (July 1994): 779–81.

Chapter 6

1. J. Fuchs and R. Milbradt, "Antioxidant Inhibition of Skin Inflammation Induced by Reactive Oxidants: Evaluation of the Redox Couple Dihydrolipoate/Lipoate," *Skin Pharmacology* 7 (1994): 278–84.

2. V. E. Kagan, A. Shvedova, E. Serbinova, S. Khan, C. Swanson, R. Powell, L. Packer, "Dihydrolipoic Acid—A Universal Antioxidant Both in the Membrane and in the Aqueous Phase. Reduction of Peroxyl, Ascorbyl and Chromanoxyl Radicals," *Biochemical Pharmacology* 44 (October 20, 1992): 1637–49.

3. Y. J. Suzuki, M. Mizuno, H. J. Tritschler, and L. Packer, "Redox Regulation of NF-kappa B DNA Binding Activity by Dihydrolipoate," *Biochemistry and Molecular Biology International* 36 (June 1995): 241–46.

4. M. Meyer, R. Schreck, and P. A. Baeuerle, "H_2O_2 and Antioxidants Have Opposite Effects on Activation of NF-kappa B and AP-1 in Intact Cells: AP-1 as Secondary Antioxidant-Responsive Factor," *EMBO Journal* 12 (May 1993): 2005–15.

5. M. Podda, M. Rallis, M. G. Traber, L. Packer, and H. I. Maibach, "Kinetic Study of Cutaneous and Subcutaneous Distribution Following Topical Application of [7,8–14C]rac-Alpha-Lipoic Acid onto Hairless Mice," *Biochemical Pharmacology* 52 (August 23, 1996): 627–33.

6. D. G. Genecov, M. Kremer, Sarah Goldberg, and Joshua Cho, "Alpha Lipoic Acid (ALA) and Scar Formation in Repaired Cleft Lips," *Transactions of the 9th International Congress on Cleft Palate and Related Craniofacial Anomalies,* Goteborg, Sweden, 25–29 June, 2001, pp. 495–99.

7. G. Filomeni, G. Rotilio, and M. R. Ciriolo, "Cell Signalling and the Glutathione Redox System," *Biochemical Pharmacology* 64 (September 2002): 1057–64.

8. P. Y. Basak, F. Gultekin, and I. Kilinc, "The Role of the Antioxidative Defense System in Papulopustular Acne," *Journal of Dermatology* 28 (March 2001): 123–27.

Index